FEMALE GENITAL PROLAPSE
and
URINARY INCONTINENCE

T0203654

FEMALE GENITAL PROLAPSE
and
URINARY INCONTINENCE

Edited by

Victor Gomel
University of British Columbia
Women's Hospital and Health Center
Vancouver, British Columbia, Canada

Bruno van Herendael
ZNA Stuivenberg
Antwerp, Belgium

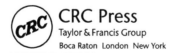

CRC Press
Taylor & Francis Group
Boca Raton London New York

CRC Press is an imprint of the
Taylor & Francis Group, an **informa** business

First published 2008 by Informa Healthcare, Inc.

Published 2019 by CRC Press
Taylor & Francis Group
6000 Broken Sound Parkway NW, Suite 300
Boca Raton, FL 33487-2742

© 2008 by Taylor & Francis Group, LLC
CRC Press is an imprint of Taylor & Francis Group, an Informa business

First issued in paperback 2019

No claim to original U.S. Government works

ISBN 13: 978-0-367-45287-2 (pbk)
ISBN 13: 978-0-8493-3656-0 (hbk)

Visit the Taylor & Francis Web site at
http://www.taylorandfrancis.com

and the CRC Press Web site at
http://www.crcpress.com

Library of Congress Cataloging-in-Publication Data

Female genital prolapse and urinary incontinence / edited by Victor Gomel,
Bruno van Herendael.
    p. ; cm.
  Includes bibliographical references and index.
  ISBN-13: 978-0-8493-3656-0 (hb : alk. paper)
  ISBN-10: 0-8493-3656-2 (hb : alk. paper) 1. Uterus–Prolapse. 2. Urinary incontinence.
3. Women–Diseases. I. Gomel, Victor. II. Herendael, Bruno van.
  [DNLM: 1. Uterine Prolapse. 2. Urinary Incontinence. WP 454 F329 2007]
  RG361.F46 2007
  616.6′2–dc22   2007025957

Foreword

When Victor Gomel and Bruno van Herendael asked me to write the foreword for *Female Genital Prolapse and Urinary Incontinence*, I felt proud and overwhelmed at the same time. The pelvic floor is the last new frontier in minimally invasive surgery for gynecologists. I have been privileged to witness this evolution over the past two decades.

As one would expect, endoscopic surgical procedures are the focus of this book, but adequate emphasis is placed on diagnostic investigations and the overriding need for a team approach to the diagnostic and therapeutic challenges of pelvic organ prolapse in the female patient. This multi-disciplinary approach is highlighted by the range of specialties represented by the authors of this book. A comprehensive array of clinical as well as radiographic investigations are discussed and reviewed. I can confidently say that *Female Genital Prolapse and Urinary Incontinence* provides a comprehensive analysis of this important clinical entity, which is important due to its prevalence and the conundrum of its pathophysiology.

The keen endoscopic surgeon will not be disappointed. The surgical procedures presented in detail are up-to-date, representing the latest minimally invasive approaches to treatment of pelvic organ prolapse. The various procedures are grouped according to the anatomical division of the anterior, middle, and posterior compartments. There is no particular bias in the selection of procedures presented. The technical description is superb and to the point. For anyone versed in minimally invasive surgery, there is little effort required to fully understand every aspect of the intervention.

Where feasible, the authors have substantiated their choice of surgical maneuvers with good science. Clinical studies are presented or reported to corroborate claims of adequacy and superiority of one method over another.

I commend the authors and editors for their professionalism and excellence in presenting their great contributions to our specialty. There is no doubt that readers will thoroughly enjoy this work as I have.

Thierry Vancaillie
Department of Obstetrics and Gynecology
University of New South Wales
Department of Endo-Gynecology
Royal Hospital for Women
Women's Health and Research
Institute of Australia
Sydney, Australia

Preface

Genital prolapse and urinary incontinence are common conditions that afflict women, especially in their postmenopausal years, and adversely affect their quality of life. Increasing life expectancy has augmented the proportion of the graying population. This, together with improved living conditions and much easier access to information, has increased the demand on the part of women for treatment of such anatomical and functional conditions that afflict them, along with their expectations of the outcomes.

In a parallel fashion, in the last 20 years we have witnessed the introduction of new surgical techniques for the treatment of both genital prolapse and urinary stress incontinence. Many of the traditional techniques have been modified and used by laparoscopic access. New and simpler techniques have been introduced to treat urinary stress incontinence. Most of these are designed to support the urethra by the placement of a strip of mesh using specially designed needles and various routes of introduction.

Dysfunction of the pelvic organs in the female is closely related to disruption of anatomy. Knowledge of anatomic changes in function of the disease is essential for successful reconstructive surgery. This prompted us to open the book with a chapter on anatomy that addresses functional changes. In the same spirit we included chapters on clinical investigation and urodynamic and radiological investigations, to define their roles in the elucidation of genital organ prolapse and urinary incontinence.

Cysto-colpo-defecography has become the keystone in the preoperative investigation of many patients, because this technique is able to pinpoint the defects in a dynamic fashion, not infrequently contradicting the clinical findings. Definitions of different abnormalities and a scoring system that allows the clarification of the extent of the problem have also been included.

In crafting the book we attempted to follow a logical sequence by dividing it into sections. Following the Introduction are three sections: the anterior, mid, and posterior segments, which represent the anatomical segments of the pelvis.

The section on the anterior segment, composed of six chapters, brings together the surgical techniques primarily used in the treatment of urinary incontinence. Data from large series are presented to compare outcomes achieved by the various available mesh techniques. Also included in this section are chapters on paraurethral treatments, which are less invasive interventions and may be further developed in the future, and computer-based artificial sphincters that provide a treatment option when all others have failed.

The section on the mid segment begins with hysterectomy, which remains the most frequently performed major gynecologic operation. This section details specific measures to prevent subsequent vault prolapse. Each of the subsequent four chapters presents a different method for the treatment of vault prolapse and lateral sidewall prolapse, aimed at obtaining a functional result. The total mesh approach is compared with the traditional suspension methods, now adapted to laparoscopic surgical access.

The section on the posterior segment has two chapters in which the classical approaches are reviewed and compared to a new laparoscopic rectal suspension technique.

In view of the many developments mentioned here, we believe that the publication of this book is timely. The 16 chapters, written by internationally recognized experts, review the pertinent aspects of the field of female genital prolapse and urinary stress incontinence, describe in detail both the more traditional and newer surgical procedures, and discuss their place and outcomes.

Victor Gomel
Bruno J. van Herendael

Contents

Contributors

Hans A. M. Brölmann Department of Obstetrics and Gynecology, VU University Medical Center, Amsterdam, The Netherlands

P. Mendes da Costa Department of Digestive and Endoscopic Surgery, CHU Brugmann, Université Libre de Bruxelles, Brussels, Belgium

Michel Degueldre Obstetrics and Gynecology Department, University Hospital St. Pierre, Brussels, Belgium

Renaud de Tayrac Groupe Hospitalier Caremeau, Service de Gynécologie-Obstétrique du Pr Mares, Nîmes, France

Kathleen D'Hauwers University Medical Center, St. Radboud, Nijmegen, The Netherlands

Jacques Donnez Department of Gynecology, Université Catholique de Louvain, Cliniques Universitaires Saint-Luc, Brussels, Belgium

Jean Bernard Dubuisson Department of Obstetrics and Gynecology, Hôpitaux Universitaires de Genève, Geneva, Switzerland

Hervé Fernandez Service de Gynécologie-Obstétrique et d'Histologie-Embryologie-Cytogénétique à orientation Biologique et Génétique de la Reproduction, Hôpital Antoine Béclère, Assistance Publique-Hôpitaux de Paris, Clamart, France

Victor Gomel Department of Obstetrics and Gynecology, Faculty of Medicine, University of British Columbia and Women's Hospital and Health Center, Vancouver, British Columbia, Canada

Danielle Hock Department of Radiology, CHC Clinique St. Joseph, Liège, Belgium

Sandrine Jacob Department of Obstetrics and Gynecology, Hôpitaux Universitaires de Genève, Geneva, Switzerland

Pascale Jadoul Department of Gynecology, Université Catholique de Louvain, Cliniques Universitaires Saint-Luc, Brussels, Belgium

Thomas Lyons Department of Obstetrics and Gynecology, Emory University, Atlanta, Georgia, U.S.A.

John R. Miklos   Atlanta UroGynecology Associates, Alpharetta, Georgia, U.S.A.

Christian Ngongang   Department of Digestive and Endoscopic Surgery, CHU Brugmann, Université Libre de Bruxelles, Brussels, Belgium

Iris Kerin Orbuch   Lenox Hill Hospital and Mount Sinai Medical Center, New York, New York, U.S.A.

Harry Reich   Wyoming Valley Health Care System, Wilkes-Barre, Pennsylvania, and Advanced Laparoscopic Surgeons, Shavertown, Pennsylvania, U.S.A.

Tamer Seckin   Department of Gynecology and Laparoscopy, Kingsbrook Jewish Medical Center, Brooklyn, New York and Lenox Hill Hospital, New York, New York, U.S.A.

Mireille Smets   Department of Gynecology, Université Catholique de Louvain, Cliniques Universitaires Saint-Luc, Brussels, Belgium

Toon P. M. Sonneville   Endoscopic Gastrointestinal Surgery, Academic Surgical Center, Antwerp, Belgium

Jean-Paul Squifflet   Department of Gynecology, Université Catholique de Louvain, Cliniques Universitaires Saint-Luc, Brussels, Belgium

Jean Vandromme   Obstetrics and Gynecology Department, University Hospital St. Pierre, Brussels, Belgium

Robrecht Van Hee   Academic Surgical Center Stuivenberg, ZNA Stuivenberg, University of Antwerp, Antwerp, Belgium

Bruno J. van Herendael   ZNA Stuivenberg, Antwerp, Belgium and Gynecology Department, Università dell'Insubria, Varese, Italy

Pieter J. Verleyen   Department of Urology, AZ Groeninge Hospital, Kortrijk, Belgium

Peter von Theobald   Department of Obstetrics, Gynecology, and Reproductive Medicine, University Hospital of Caen, Caen, France

Jean-Marie Wenger   Department of Obstetrics and Gynecology, Hôpitaux Universitaires de Genève, Geneva, Switzerland

Jean Jacques Wyndaele   Department of Urology, Faculty of Medicine, University of Antwerp, Antwerp, Belgium

Part I: Introduction

————————————— **1** —————————————

Dynamic Anatomy of the Pelvic Floor

Michel Degueldre and Jean Vandromme

*Obstetrics and Gynecology Department, University Hospital St. Pierre,
Brussels, Belgium*

Bruno J. van Herendael

*ZNA Stuivenberg, Antwerp, Belgium and Gynecology Department,
Università dell'Insubria, Varese, Italy*

INTRODUCTION

Before taking off it would be interesting to know how to land.
—Arnaud Wattiez

Multiple challenges await the surgeon who operates on the pelvic area. Although specific anatomical landmarks define the limits of the operating field as in any other surgical field, very specific situations exist in this area:

- Nerve-sparing surgery becomes mandatory to retain the function of the different organs.
- Pressure gradients in the different compartments play an important role in the postoperative success rate for suspension surgery.
- The anatomical and functional interaction of the organs is very important to guarantee normal function of both the sexual and voiding aspects of daily life.

These factors make pelvic surgery in the female a challenge. A thorough knowledge is necessary not only of pelvic anatomy, vascular-nervous-muscular-ligamental-fascial-virtual and physical spaces (foramina), and bony structures, but also of the mechanical forces and physiological processes.

Pelvic surgeons have to realize that there exist two different anatomies: the one that is described in anatomy books and observed in cadaver dissections and the one that is encountered during surgery. We need to find specific solutions for the specific patient.

It would be ideal to have a three-dimensional virtual reality picture of the patient's anatomy to properly assess the condition before making surgical decisions (Figs. 1–3).

Virtual reality imaging is not yet available, but the spiral CT scan provides detailed imaging (Figs. 4–7). Computer software programs provide the capability to produce moving images from the sequence of still pictures. By sailing through the tissues the viewer gets the impression of a virtual reality image.

The aim of this chapter is to provide a pictorial description of the female pelvis combining anatomical, physiological, and functional data.

The pelvis of the human female is divided into three functional entities: (*i*) the anterior compartment; (*ii*) the mid compartment; and (*iii*) the posterior compartment (Fig. 8).

The Anterior Compartment

Bone: Starting front to back this compartment contains: the pubic bone, consisting of the superior pubic ramus, the pectineal line (pectin Ossis pubis) ending median in the pubic tubercle, the crista obturatoria, the inferior pubic ramus and the ramus of the ischial bone.

Foramina: The main foramen in the anterior compartment is the obturator foramen delineated anteriorly by the superior pubic ramus and the inferior pubic ramus. This entity is sealed by the obturator membrane and leaves

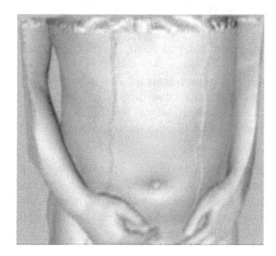

Figure 1   This view is similar to what the physician would see looking at the patient. *Source*: Courtesy of J. Marescaux IRCAD/EITS University of Strasbourg, France.

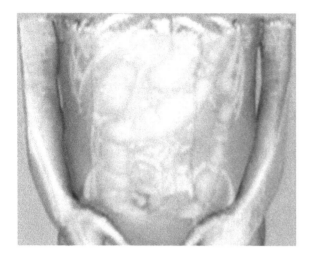

Figure 2 The images, obtained by spiral CT scan of the same patient are treated by computer subtraction of elements to visualize the internal organs. *Source*: Courtesy of J. Marescaux IRCAD/EITS University of Strasbourg, France.

openings superior and lateral under the superior ramus: the obturator channels.

Fascia: These include the urogenital fascia (inferior and superior fascia diaphragmatis urogenitalis), which incorporate the median and lateral pubovesical ligaments anteriorly; the vesicocervical fascial fibers (pubocervical or urogenital); and the tendineus arch of the levator ani muscle. The fascia is the border between the anterior and mid compartments.

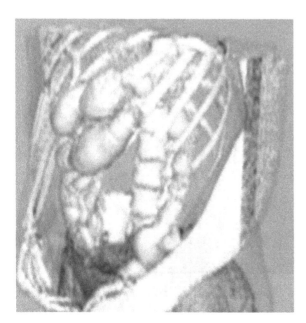

Figure 3 The computer subtraction of elements is now complete, leaving only the study objects, the colon, and the bony elements to be considered. These images can be rotated to visualize the subject from different angles. *Source*: Courtesy of J. Marescaux IRCAD/EITS University of Strasbourg, France.

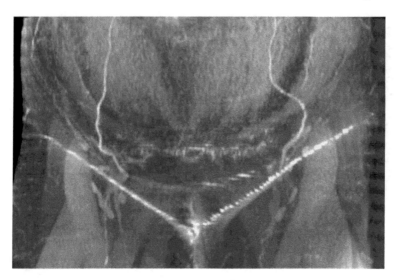

Figure 4   Spiral CT scan image of the frontal view of the lower abdomen. Note the course of the epigastric arteries from the inguinal region to the umbilicus.

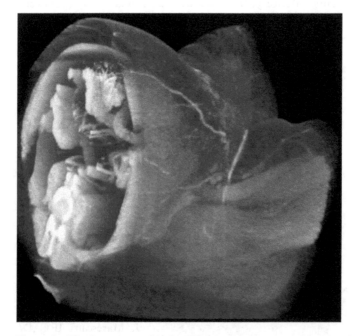

Figure 5   The image may be tilted (in the transverse position here) to visualize the pelvic area in the conventional way.

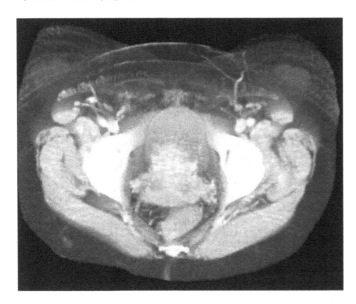

Figure 6 In this image, the lower pelvic area is seen with the bladder in front of the uterus. The bony structures of the pelvis are seen along with the different muscular structures. Note the blood vessels at the level of the inguinal canal, the femoral artery and vein, and the vena saphena magna running down the inner aspect of the leg.

Ligaments: The symphysis pubis with the superior pubic ligament and Cooper's ligaments over the superior pubic ramus are the more important landmarks for the surgeon. The other ligaments encountered when moving from anterior to posterior are: the median and lateral pubovesical ligaments, the inguinal ligament (Poupart's), and the round ligament over its most distal part in the inguinal canal. There are also the arcuate pubic ligament and the transverse perineal ligament.

Muscles: Laterally from the exterior toward the center are the obturator muscle and the anterior aspect of the levator ani muscle. Anteriorly and superiorly are the layers of the rectus abdominal muscle. The deepest part of the female pelvis is closed, anterior by part of a transverse muscle layer surrounding the genital hiatus composed of the ischio-cavernosus, laterally and the bulbo-spongiosus delineating the vagina. Both muscles rest on and are part of the deep transverse perineal muscle.

Nerves: Knowledge of the location and function of the various neural structures and their preservation are essential for the successful outcome of the surgical intervention. The neurological structures of this compartment are: the femoral nerve, the ilio-inguinal nerve, superficial and deep branches of the perineal nerve, the perineal branch of the posterior femoral cutaneous nerve, and the pudendal nerve (somatic) from the sacral plexus (S2–S4).

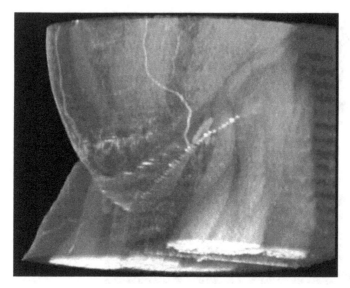

Figure 7 Once the coronal view is analyzed the image can be tilted to a transverse position. The lower body is now turned from the frontal view toward the side by 20°. Note the course of the epigastric artery.

Both sensory and somatic fibers from the lower vagina and the perineum accompany the pudendal nerve. The urinary bladder and the lower ureter are serviced by pre- and post-ganglionic sympathetic and parasympathetic fibers.

- Parasympathetic from S2-S3-S4 (vesical plexus) responsible for transudation at the vaginal level and erection at the level of the clitoris.
- Sympathetic from L1 to L2: the plexus hypogastricus superior ending in the nervus hypogastricus to form the plexus hypogastricus inferior and the plexus uterovaginalis (plexus of Frankenhäuser) terminating in the nervus vaginalis. The main action of these sympathetic fibers is contraction.
- Somatomotoric and somatosensitive: from S2 to S4 the nervus pudendus ending at this level in the nervus dorsalis clitoridis and the nervi labiales posteriores. The main action of the nerve fibers is contraction.

Vessels: Superior and inferior vesical arteries and veins (branches respectively of the umbilical artery and vein and the middle rectal artery and vein) supply the bladder. The vagina gets its blood supply through the vaginal artery and vein (branches of the internal iliac artery and vein). The anterior compartment also contains the inferior epigastric artery and vein (branches of the external iliac artery and vein), a structure best avoided during laparoscopic entry.

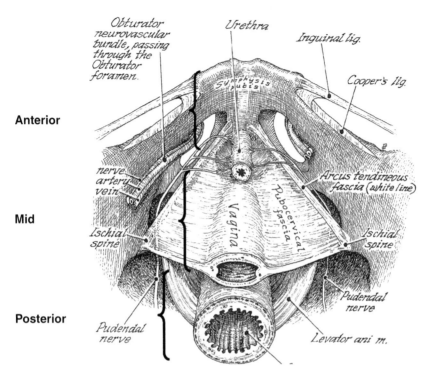

Figure 8 The anatomy of the three compartments of the pelvis viewed from above. *Source*: Reprinted by permission from Hulka and Reich, *Textbook of Laparoscopy*.

Lymphatic structures: The most important lymphatic structures of this compartment are the inguinal nodes; the most distal of these are situated under the inguinal (Poupart's) ligament.

Organs: The organs in this compartment include the clitoris, the labia, the bladder, the urethra, and the distal portion of the ureter.

Spaces: The space of Retzius is the retropubic space bordered anteriorly by the pelvic bone, posterior by the endopelvic fascia (urogenital, pubocervical, or pelvic fascia), covering the bladder and the urethra, and on the lateral borders by the obturator muscle.

All of these structures have their own specific, necessary function of which the surgeon should be well aware. It is extremely important for any surgeon to realize that destructive surgery on the organs usually means destructive surgery on the local nerves and their interactivity, and therefore will result in loss of perception and function after even very simple but ill-executed surgery. Figures 9 and 10 provide a clear view of the anterior compartment, including the symphysis pubis, bony structures, muscles, Cooper's ligaments,

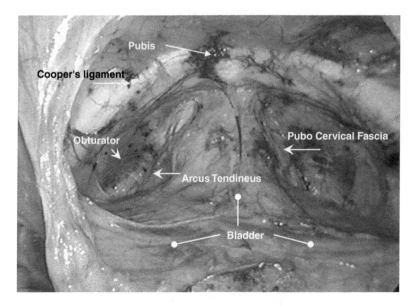

Figure 9 Laparoscopic view of the anterior compartment of the pelvis and the space of Retzius.

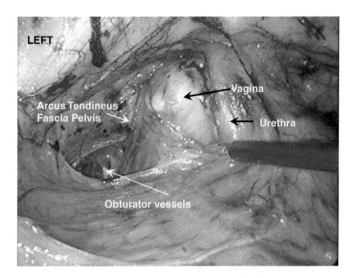

Figure 10 Laparoscopic view of the left side of the anterior compartment of the pelvis. The vagina, white shiny aspect of the pubovesical fascia, and obturator vessels are seen after carefully freeing the area from the overlying bladder seen behind the instrument.

and the bladder. It is evident that the vessels and the nerves are difficult to distinguish despite the magnification offered by the laparoscope, hence the need for the surgeon to be careful.

The Mid Compartment

Bones: From high up anterior toward deep posterior: the iliac bone with the spina iliaca anterior inferior and further dorsal the spina iliaca anterior superior at the beginning of the crista iliaca, the arcuate line, the corpus ossis ischii, the tuber ischiadicum and finally the spina ischiadica.

Foramina: On the anterior side, the posterior aspect of the obturator foramen, on the posterior side the ischiadic foramen. The greater sciatic foramen and the lesser sciatic foramen are in fact one large opening divided into two by the ischial spine and the sacrospinous ligament.

Fascia: The inferior and superior sheet of the urogenital fascia is called pubo-vesico-vaginal fascia; it commences in the anterior compartment and attaches to the ischial spine in the middle compartment. The posterior and lower aspect of the urogenital facia is called the recto vesical fascia (Denonvilliers fascia). There are many components to this large fascial structure. It must be realized that fascial structures do descend from the lateral pelvic walls and unify in the centre of the pelvis, to form a strong functional entity.

Ligaments: The sacrospinal ligament and the sacrotuberous ligaments are the most prominent in the mid section. The arcus tendineus of the pelvic fascia runs on both sides of the hiatus genitalis, from anterior to posterior, originating at the medial pubovesical ligament and the vesicocervical fascia to unify with the uterosacral ligament. The arcus tendineus of the levator ani muscle is situated on the pelvic wall parallel to the arcus tendineus of the pelvic fascia, some 2–3 cm lateral to the former and forms the border with the internal obturator muscle on the pelvic side wall. Inter-digitizing fibers of the superior fascia of the pelvic diaphragm run, as part of the mid-section ligaments, between the vagina and the rectum (Fig. 10).

Muscles: The Pubococcygeus and the Puborectalis muscles, in the middle compartment, are part of the levator ani muscular complex. The pubo-coccygeus runs from the Os Pubis towards the Os Coxys in the midline encircling the hiatus genitalis and attaches to the arcus tendineus musculi levator ani on the lateral side of the pelvis (Fig. 11). The deep transverse perineal muscle runs from side-to-side deep in the pelvis encircling the vagina. The superficial transverse perineal muscle runs from the side wall to the central tendon of the perineum just under the vagina. The obturator internus muscle covers the lateral and side aspect over the obturator membrane.

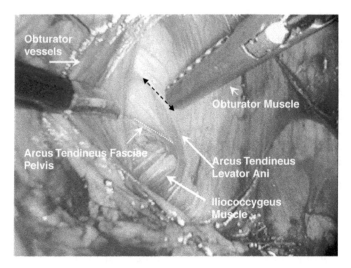

Figure 11 Laparoscopic view of the lateral aspect of the mid compartment of the female pelvis (right side).

Nerves: Nerve plexuses are frequently composed of nerve fibers with different potentials. This is especially the case in the mid compartment of the pelvis. The right and left hypogastric nerve bundles, originating from the superior hypogastric plexus, are sympathetic nerves that form the inferior hypogastric plexus. These are the main nervous structures. According to the function we can subdivide into:

- Parasympathetic: S2 to S4 nervi pelvici splanchnici, nervi erigentes of the plexus sacralis to the tube, the uterus and the vagina and their function is mainly vasodilatation.
- Sympathetic:
  - Th10 to Th12 plexus mesentericus superior and the plexus renalis to form the plexus ovaricus. The main function here is vaso-constriction.
  - L1 to L2 The plexus hypogastricus to form the nervus hypogastricus to form the plexus hypogastricus inferior to end in the plexus utero vaginalis (plexus of Lee and Frankenhäuser). The main function is contraction at the level of the tube, the uterus and the vagina.

Vessels: There are numerous vascular structures in this compartment. The common iliac vessels, artery and vein, originating from the aorta and vena cava respectively; the external iliac artery and vein that give rise to the deep circumflex iliac vessels, the inferior epigastric artery and vein, and the internal iliac artery and vein. The internal iliac artery and vein are the source of mid-pelvic vessels that include the uterine artery and vein, the vaginal artery and vein on a truncus communis with the uterine artery, the middle rectal artery and vein, and the internal pudendal artery and vein. The last vessels give rise to the anterior rectal artery and vein. Branches of the internal iliac artery and vein that start from the posterior compartment of the pelvis but are players in the mid-pelvis include the obturator artery and vein and the umbilical artery and vein. The ovarian arteries and veins are from a different origin as they originate from higher in the body; the right ovarian artery and vein from the aorta and vena cava, respectively, and the left ovarian artery from the aorta but the left ovarian vein from the left renal vein.

Lymphatic structures: The mid compartment contains the obturator, the medial (inferior) external iliac, and the lateral (superior) external iliac nodes. The internal iliac nodes are situated alongside the internal iliac artery and the vessels originating from it. The paracervical section of the broad ligament is another area where lymph nodes are found that are part of the internal iliac node chain.

Organs: The organs contained in this compartment include the uterus, tubes and the ovaries in the transverse plane; the ureter, in the antero-posterior axis, running from the pelvic brim towards the bladder on the lower part of the pelvis; and the vagina that communicates the exterior of the body with the internal genitalia.

Ligaments: Two major ligaments support the uterus; they are the uterosacral ligaments, between the lower posterior part of the uterus and the sacrum, in the antero-posterior axis of the pelvis; and the broad ligaments (ligamentum latum) which incorporate the Cardinal or Mackenrodt's ligaments. The latter consists of a densification of tissues under the uterine artery and veins between the upper part of the uterine cervix and the pelvic bone. Part of the broad ligament is also the proper ovarian ligament (ligamentum ovarii proprium)—between the lateral part of the uterine fundus and the hilus of the ovary. Another part is the ligamentum rotundum teres, or round ligament commencing on the uterine fundus near the insertion of the tube, and going laterally and inferiorly to the inguinal canal. The broad ligaments are situated laterally and extend on both sides from the uterus towards the lateral pelvic walls. It is a double layer structure consisting of three peritoneal meso's: the funicular meso, the meso-salpinx and the meso-ovarium. The funicular meso covers the round ligament that joins the uterine cornu to the inguinal canal. When opened it allows access to the paravesical space. The meso-salpinx extends from the fallopian tube on the upper, anterior aspect, laterally and posteriorly to the infundibulo pelvic ligament. It contains the infra-ovarian and tubal branches of the ovarian vessels and the infra tubal neural plexus. Close to the uterus the border of the meso-salpinx becomes the ovarian ligament (ligamentum ovarium proprium). The meso-ovarium contains the ovarian vessels and the nerves.

Space: In the mid compartment there are four spaces that can be identified and play a role in pelvic surgery.

1. The paravesical space is located between the uterus and the bladder in the anterior part of the broad ligament. It is entered between the umbilical artery and the external iliac vessels. The floor consists of the levator ani muscle and the ilio-pubic muscle. The predominant features of this space are the obturator nerve and the obturator artery and vein in the fossa obturatoria. The obturator nerve runs towards the obturator foramen originating from the plexus lumbosacralis.
2. The para-rectal space is located in the posterior lower aspect of the broad ligament, between the rectum and the posterior limits of the cervix (the components of the para-cervix) under the uterosacral ligament. The piriform muscle forms the lateral border and lateral rectal ligament the posterior border. The levator ani muscle forms the base of this space.
3. The pouch of Douglas consists of the peritoneal fold confined by the uterosacral ligaments on the sides, the uterine cervix anteriorly and the anterior margin of the rectum posterior.
4. The recto vaginal space or septum is limited posterior by the rectum, laterally by the uterosacral ligaments, anteriorly by the vagina, inferiorly by the levator ani muscle and anal sphincter and superiorly by the peritoneal layer of the pouch of Douglas.

The Posterior Compartment

As evident from Figures 12–17, the border between the mid and posterior compartments is an arbitrary rather than a functional entity. Most of the arteries, veins, nerves and organs run from the posterior to the mid compartment.

Bones: The sacrum is the most prominent bony feature and forms the posterior border of this compartment. The fifth lumbar vertebral body forms its upper and the coccyx its inferior border. The iliac bones that forms the iliac fossa encloses the compartment laterally; the lower two-thirds are taken up by the greater sciatic foramen and the lesser sciatic foramen.

Foramina: The main spaces are the greater and lesser sciatic foramina delineated anteriorly, laterally and superiorly by the body of the iliac bone. The ischial spine (Fig. 18) and the sacrospinal ligament divide the greater from the lesser sciatic foramen. The lesser foramen is delineated anteriorly by the body of the ischial bone up to the ischial tuberosity. The posterior border is the lateral side of the sacrum. The greater foramen is bordered by the os ileum, the os ischiadicum and the sacrum its lower border is the sacrospinal ligament.

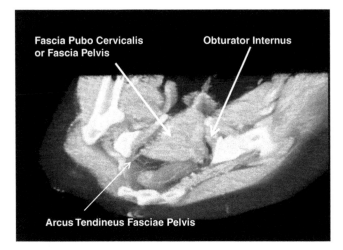

Figure 12 The anterior part of the mid compartment of the pelvis, in a coronary view, with the landmarks running in a sagittal plane as seen through the computer analysis of a spiral CT scanning image.

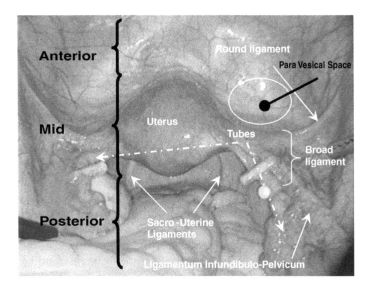

Figure 13 Panoramic view of the three compartments of the pelvis viewed with the laparoscope. The dominant organ in the mid-pelvis is the uterus. The infundibulo-pelvic ligaments contain the collateral circulation to the uterus. The tubes have been secured with Hulka-Clemens clips as means of definitive contraception. The small cyst on the right is a para-salpingeal cyst. The paravesical space is highlighted with a white circle. Note that the fallopian tubes and the ovaries are not bound to one compartment, nor are the infundibulo pelvic ligaments and the ureter, which is not visible on this picture.

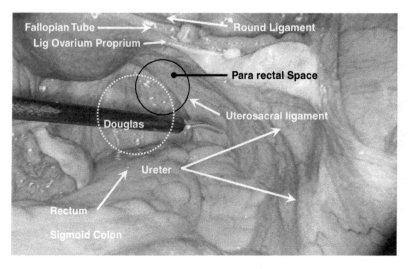

Figure 14 Laparoscopic view of the mid-pelvis: the uterosacral ligament, the ovarian ligament, and part of the round ligament are seen. The broad ligament runs from the uterosacral ligament towards the pelvic side wall in the transverse axis of the pelvis. The location of the para-rectal space is indicated with a black circle and the pouch of Douglas with a dotted white circle.

Ligaments: From top to bottom there are: the *ilio lumbar ligament*, running from the pelvic bone to the lumbar vertebral body; the *anterior sacro iliac ligament* between the sacrum and the iliac fossa; the *posterior sacro iliac ligament* between the same structures forming the posterior border of the greater sciatic foramen; the *sacro spinous ligament* between the sacrum and the ischial spine; and the *sacro tuberous ligament* between the sacrum and the ischial tuberosity at the bottom of the pelvis and providing support to the tendon of the long head of the biceps femoris muscle. *The anterior sacro coccygeal ligament* that runs from the sacrum towards the coccyx in the center of the posterior compartment. The tendinous arch of the levator ani muscle runs on the sidewall to stop at the insertion of the muscle at the ischial spine. The deepest posterior is the anococcygeal ligament running from the fibers of the anal muscle towards the os coccyx.

Muscles: From top to bottom there are the piriform muscle, the coccygeus muscle, the ilio coccygeus part of the levator ani, the pubococcygeus part of the levator ani, and the puborectalis part of the levator ani. All these muscles are attached to the tendinous arch of the levator ani. The external anal sphincter and anterior the superficial transverse perineal muscle are the most distal muscles of the pelvic floor.

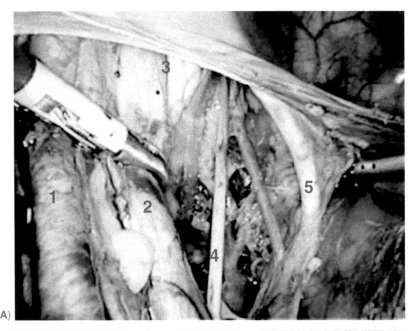

(A)

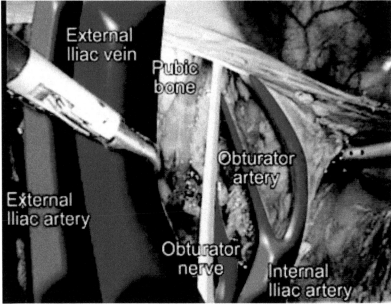

(B)

Figure 15 (A) Laparoscopic view of the left external iliac artery and vein (**1**), the ramus of the pubic bone (**2**), the obturator nerve (**3**), the obturator vein and artery (**4**) and the obliterated artery (**5**). (B) Computer filling of the same view. *Source*: Courtesy of Fabio Ghezzi Varese.

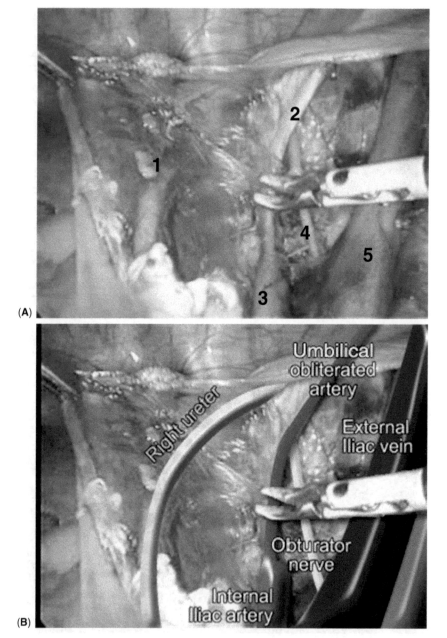

Figure 16 (**A**) Laparoscopic view of the right side of the mid-pelvis after the dissection of the obturator fossa. The right ureter (**1**), the obliterated umbilical artery (**2**), ending in the internal iliac artery (**3**), the obturator nerve (**4**), and the external iliac vein (**5**). (**B**) Computer filling of the same view. *Source*: Courtesy of Fabio Ghezzi Varese.

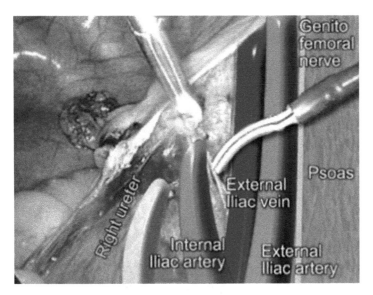

Figure 17   Another computer-enhanced view of the right obturator fossa and the side wall of the border between the mid and posterior pelvic compartments to demonstrate the position of the genito femoral nerve. *Source*: Courtesy of Fabio Ghezzi Varese.

Nerves: The sensory fibers of the rectal plexus accompany the sympathetic fibers via the pelvic plexus. Motor fibers go via the pudendal nerve (somatic) that also innervates the perineum. Sensory fibers accompany the somatic fibers via the pudendal nerve S2, 3 and 4. The pudendal nerve also innervates the anal region via the inferior rectal nerve and the perineum via the perineal nerve. The zone around the ano coccygeal ligament is innervated by the ano coccygeal nerves. The genito femoral nerve runs on the anterior side of the psoas muscle and divides into the femoral and the genital branch. The femoral nerve lies very deep on the border between the psoas and the levator muscles.

Vessels: The vascular structures of this compartment include:

1. The external iliac artery and vein that run along the lateral pelvic wall; after the separation of the internal iliac artery and vein and they give rise to the inferior epigastric artery and vein.
2. The internal iliac artery and vein; these give rise successively, to the obturator artery and vein to the patent parts of the umbilical artery and veins, the uterine artery and vein, the vaginal artery and vein and the middle rectal artery and vein. The inferior vesical arteries and veins originate from the patent part of the umbilical artery.

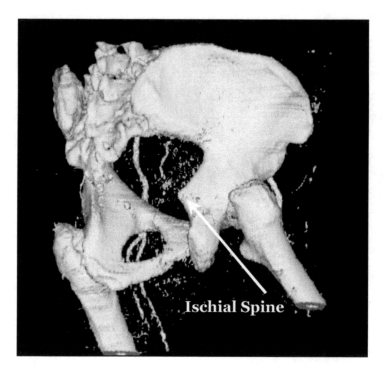

Ischial Spine

Figure 18   After subtraction of the muscles and most of the soft tissues, the CT scan of the bones gives a good idea of the position in space of the ischial spine.

There are also the ovarian arteries and veins that lay within the infundibulo-pelvic ligament (the right ovarian vein originates from the vena cava, while the left from the left renal vein); the middle sacral artery and vein, usually located in the mid-sacral region; the superior rectal artery which runs alongside and to the left of the middle sacral vessels; the artery and vein iliolumbalis, which are not that well known, also run alongside the middle sacral artery and vein (Figs. 19–24).

Lymphatic structures: These include the mid sacral (promontory) nodes located in the region of the promontory of the sacrum. The lateral sacral nodes situated below and lateral to the mid sacral nodes, common iliac nodes located immediately lateral to the mid sacral nodes, between the common iliac vein and artery. There is also the lateral aortic of lumbar nodes; these are in fact outside of the pelvis, yet of great importance in oncological surgery.

Organs: The rectum and the sigmoid colon are the main organs in the posterior compartment of the pelvis.

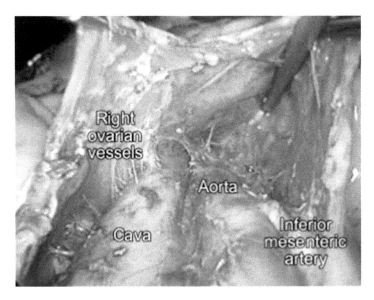

Figure 19 Laparoscopic view of the main vessels in the lower abdomen immediately above the pelvis: aorta and the vena cava and the origin of the ovarian vessels. *Source*: Courtesy of Fabio Ghezzi Varese.

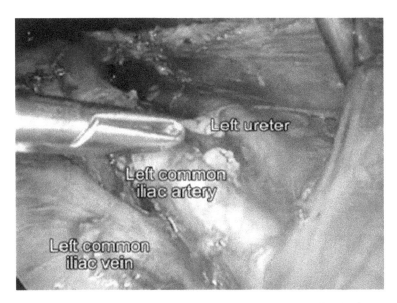

Figure 20 Laparoscopic view of the structures on the left side just under the bifurcation of the aorta and the vena cava. *Source*: Courtesy of Fabio Ghezzi Varese.

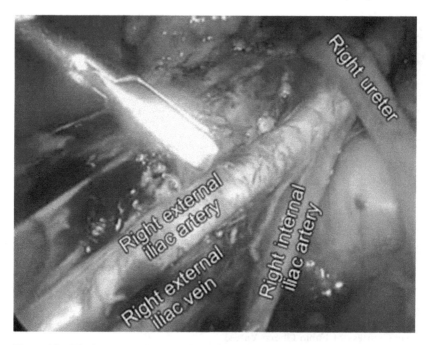

Figure 21 The laparoscopic view of the region below the division of the internal and external iliac vessels. Note the position of the ureter. *Source*: Courtesy of Fabio Ghezzi Varese.

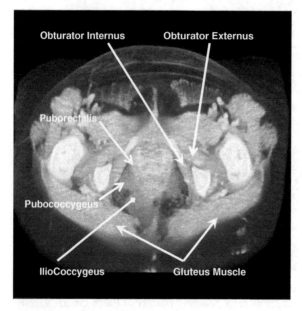

Figure 22 CT scan image of the muscles in the posterior and the mid compartments of the lower aspect of the pelvic floor.

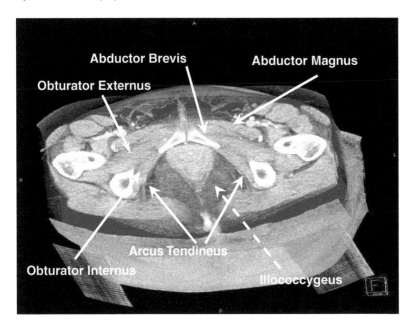

Figure 23 Gray-scale CT scan with the different muscles and the arcus tendineus of the ilio coccygeus muscle.

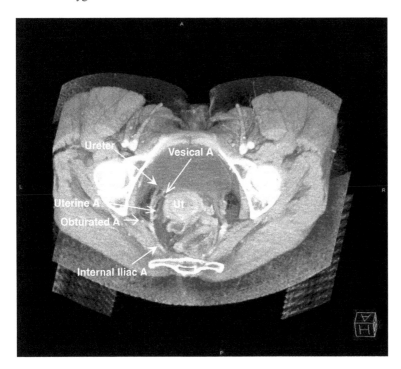

Figure 24 Gray-scale CT scan of the posterior and mid compartments illustrating the vessels in relation to the ureter.

BIBLIOGRAPHY

Donnez J, Nisolle M. An Atlas of Operative Laparoscopy and Hysteroscopy, 2nd edn. New York: The Parthenon Publishing Group; 2001, 33–45.

Frank H. Netter, 8th edn. Ciba-Geigy Corporation Summit: NJ, USA; 1995, 334–94.

Hulka JF and Reich H. *Textbook of Laparoscopy*, 3rd ed. Philadelphia: WB Saunders; 1998, 317–79.

Putz R, Pabst R. Atlas of Human Anatomy: Sobotta, Part 2. Houten, The Netherlands: Bohn Stafleu Van Loghum; 1994, 130–259.

2

History and Clinical Investigations: Patient Complaints in Perspective

Hans A. M. Brölmann

Department of Obstetrics and Gynecology, VU University Medical Center, Amsterdam, The Netherlands

INTRODUCTION

A pelvic floor disorder is defined by one of the following conditions: pelvic organ prolapse (POP) and incontinence for urine or feces. As the prevalence of pelvic floor defects increases with age, the problem will grow more important in the aging population of the West. The prevalence of pelvic floor defects has a wide range between studies because different criteria (numerator) and varying populations (denominator) are used. In a population-based study (1) a prevalence of POP of 3.9% was found, increasing with age. The lifetime risk to undergo prolapse surgery at the age of 60 is 5% and increases to 11% by the age of 80 (2). Estimates in literature concerning urinary stress incontinence vary from 4% to 50% (3). Fecal incontinence increases with age, and the prevalence in the general community is reported to be 2.2% in all age groups (63% of the patients are female) (4).

To assess the severity of POP a careful medical history is necessary, followed by a pelvic examination. According to all conditions requiring surgery, the surgeon is obliged to obtain as many objective data as possible concerning the pelvic floor defect and the correlated symptoms. Some symptoms are specific to the site of the prolapse. The pelvic floor anatomy is divided into three compartments: the anterior compartment with the urethrocele and cystocele, the middle or apical compartment with the uterine descent, and the enterocele and the posterior compartment with the rectocele and perineal descent (5). A substantial progress has been made in recent years concerning the process of getting objective data. In 1996, the International Continence Society (ICS) has proposed the POP-quantification score (6) to replace the arbitrary scoring systems available and used in the past. This scoring system has been accepted, though not yet widely implemented. At the same time the translation of the symptoms into a POP-quantification (POP-Q) score has been studied extensively (7). Both methods of assessing genital prolapse, separately and/or in combination will be addressed in this chapter in order to offer a more solid base for the clinician to manage POP as correctly as possible.

SYMPTOMS

It has been generally assumed that the severity of symptoms caused by the genital prolapse depends on the site and stage of the prolapse (8). In general, symptoms tend to occur relatively late in the process of POP. However, there is substantial overlap of symptoms at the different prolapse sites. In order to evaluate if specific complaints are correlated to the severity of the prolapse, correlation of the symptoms with the POP-Q stage was studied by Swift et al. (9). In a general female population attending the gynecologic clinic for preventive female health care, the correlations between the standardized POP-Q score and the seven following complaints: "falling out," visualization of bulge, urinary incontinence, fecal or flatus incontinence, "splinting to defecate," "low back pain" and "groin pain" have been studied. The last two complaints did not demonstrate a correlation with the stage of the prolapse, therefore those were considered specific. The patients with a prolapse exceeding stage III (>1 cm beyond hymen) answered positive on more than two out of five questions, in which two of the three considered the prolapse as "bothersome." In stage 0 (no prolapse) a positive answer was received in 0.27 times. These findings make a causal relationship of the abovementioned complaints with prolapse likely. Constipation is reported as frequent as 67% in prolapse patients, has no relationship with the severity of the prolapse and might be an etiologic factor in the development of prolapse rather than a result (10).

To know whether a specific symptom can be attributed to a prolapse as such or more specific to the anterior, apical or posterior compartment, the correlation between symptoms and POP-Q stage was studied according to site by Ellerkmann et al. (10) and by Mouritsen and Larsen (11). Urinary stress incontinence is inversely related to the stage of cystocele; however, there is a positive correlation with the difficulty of voiding. This can be explained by the increased kinking of the urethra in the higher stages of cystocele. Incomplete evacuation of stools or the need of digital manipulation ("splinting the vagina") is only related to the stage of rectocele. Impairment of sexual life seems mostly related to apical (enterocele and uterine or vaginal vault prolapse) and anterior prolapse. A lump at the introitus (visualization of a bulge) is seen more frequently in cases of the combination of anterior and posterior prolapse (11). Complaints attributed to the different sites of prolapse and their sometimes widely ranging frequencies are listed in Table 1.

A problem in taking the medical history might be under-reporting by the patients caused by their embarrassment, undermining the reliability. This concerns, in particular, urinary or fecal incontinence. Among women

Table 1 Frequency of POP-Related Complaints in Symptomatic Women Seeking Help for Presumed POP

	% Ellerkmann et al. (10)	% Mouritsen and Larsen (11)
General		
Lower abdominal pressure[a]	63	–
Pelvic heaviness[a]	56	72
Pelvic discomfort[a]	58	–
Visualization of bulge[a]	43	70
Anterior compartment		
Urinary incontinence[a]	73	48
Stress incontinence only[a]	10	27
Difficulty emptying bladder[a]	49	54
Sensation of incomplete voiding	62	–
Hesitancy[a]	34	
Weak/prolonged flow[a]	56	–
Intermittent flow[a]	44	–
Post-void dribbling[a]	55	–
Require position change[a]	40	–
Urgency[a]	–	44
Frequency[a]	–	45
Nocturia (>2/night)[a]	–	12
Rec. cystitis (>2/year)[a]	–	8
Apical compartment		
Impairment of sex life	57	35–57
Posterior compartment		
Constipation[a]	67	19
Dyschesia[a]	41	–
Digital manipulation	24	23
Fecal or flatus incontinence	31	34

Note: The symptoms are listed according to the most likely prolapse site associated with them.
[a]Site specificity not demonstrated in Ellerkmann et al. results.
Abbreviation: POP, pelvic organ prolapse.

with incontinence, this symptom is often perceived as a normal part of aging and the under-reporting can be considered as a coping mechanism. An active approach is warranted and questionnaires, delivered to and filled out by the patients prior to the history-taking by the physician, may be helpful in encouraging openness. According to Table 1 the many symptoms that are reported in relation to prolapse are briefly discussed.

GENERAL SYMPTOMS

The patient may have general complaints that are independent of the anatomic site of the prolapse. These are generally mechanical by nature and a consequence of herniation of the pelvic floor. The descent of the uterus and/or vagina causes a sense of "falling out." Sometimes a bulge or "lump" may be visible. These complaints may be described as pelvic discomfort, pelvic heaviness or lower abdominal pressure. In the study of Ellerkmann (10) of 237 patients seeking medical help for prolapse-related symptoms, these complaints occurred in 43% to 63% of the cases. The strongest correlation with POP-Q stage had the "visualizing of the bulge" (0.40–0.44 Kendall's τ), which can be considered very specific for prolapse.

ANTERIOR COMPARTMENT

The relaxation of the anterior wall results in an urethrocele (urethra and bladder neck) and a cystocele. While an urethrocele results in stress incontinence, a cystocele without descent of the bladder neck causes obstructed micturition.

According to the ICS, urinary incontinence as a medical disorder is "a condition in which involuntary loss of urine is a social or hygienic problem and is objectively demonstrable" (12). In the case of urethrocele, also referred to as a hyper-mobile urethra, the musculus compressor urethra as a part of the musculus pubococcygeus cannot effectively close the urethra during the contraction of the muscle. Also, the urethral sphincter and possibly the transmission of abdominal pressure play a role. During straining (coughing, sneezing, laughing) involuntary loss of urine develops. This is a phenomenon known as urinary stress incontinence (USI). It has been difficult to define the degree, quantity and frequency of urine loss necessary to qualify it as pathology. A well-established classification of (stress) incontinence is not available. Incontinence has been reported at a frequency of 26% at some stage during their lives in a study of randomly chosen women aged 30 to 59 years, and 14% of the women perceived incontinence to be a social or a hygienic problem. It is important to rule out signs of an overactive bladder (OAB) such as frequency, urgency and urge incontinence, as it will reduce success rate of subsequent incontinence surgery. Urge incontinence constitutes 10% to 15% in younger women, and

30% to 40% in older women. Stress incontinence tends to be more common in women younger than 65 years. In patients older than 65 years, urge incontinence and mixed (i.e., urge and stress) incontinence is more common. In the presence of urinary incontinence, serious sexual problems may develop. In a multiple regression model, urinary incontinence was significantly associated with low libido [odds ratio (OR) 1.96], vaginal dryness (OR 2.11) and dysparoenia (OR 2.04), independent of age, educational attainment and race (13).

In case of POP-Q stage III–IV (see later in this chapter) of the uterus or the bladder (cystocele), the urethra may kink and micturition will be obstructed (Fig. 1). This causes symptoms such as hesitancy, weak/prolonged flow, necessity to change position (leaning forward) to pass urine, that are specific to prolapse of the anterior compartment and do rarely occur in prolapse of the posterior compartment (10). Sometimes the patient manually redresses the anterior wall during micturition in order to void freely. A possible health hazard is the recurring cystitis that may result from repeated incomplete voiding.

Apical compartment prolapse in this compartment comprises uterine descent, vaginal vault prolapse and entero(culdo)cele. There are different views on the correlation between prolapse and the impairment of sexual life of the individual patient. Such a correlation is demonstrated for the posterior and anterior compartment (Kendall's τ: 0.28–0.30), but most clearly

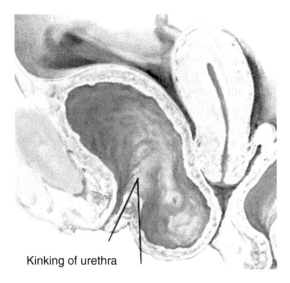

Kinking of urethra

Figure 1 In this longitudinal image of the pelvis a large cystocele is shown and kinking of the urethra, which causes incomplete emptying of the bladder. *Source*: With permission from Frank Netter, Ciba Atlas.

for the mid (apical) compartment (Kendall's τ: 0.43) (10). However, if there is no incontinence present, no such correlation seems to exist and age appears the predominant factor in predicting sexual function (13,14). Sometimes loss of tight fitting, "looseness," during sexual intercourse is presented as a complaint. Usually this is prompted by the sexual partner. The symptom may be more psychogenic than anatomic in nature (8). Marital counseling or pelvic floor muscle exercise may make surgery redundant.

The posterior zone symptom complex as described by Petros (15) regards actually the enterocele and comprises: frequency, urgency, nocturia, pelvic pain and abnormal voiding. These complaints may be caused by the stretching of the autonomous nervous fibers running through the sacrouterine ligament. Although longitudinal data are lacking in operated patients the presence of frequency (43%), urgency (46%) and pelvic pain (heaviness) (54%) in patients with enterocele is confirmed in the study by Mouritsen and Larsen (11).

POSTERIOR COMPARTMENT

Prolapse in the posterior compartment contains rectocele and perineal descent, mostly because of obstetrical lacerations. The main complaint is the inability to expel the feces that are stuck in the rectocele. Digital splinting of the vagina is necessary to open the bowel and is considered to be specific for posterior compartment prolapse (11). Firm stools because of constipation will only pass with great difficulty and softening the stools is mandatory and preferred to surgery in case of a mild rectocele. Constipation is not related to the site of the prolapse and may play an etiologic role in posterior compartment prolapse. The symptom dyschesia (painful and difficult stools) is related to this problem with evacuation. Perineal descent may be a crucial factor in the development of the symptoms of the posterior compartment as the combination of rectocele and perineal descent causes more symptoms than rectocele alone (16).

In the two referred studies of symptomatic POP-patients (11,10) incontinence for flatus or stools was reported in 34% and in 31%, respectively, of the patients. It is remarkable that no significant correlation was demonstrated with the site of the prolapse. Incontinence for flatus did occur more frequently (32%) than for solid stools (11%) (11).

QUALITY-OF-LIFE AND PELVIC FLOOR DYSFUNCTION

Health has been defined by the World Health Organization (WHO) (17) according to their handbook of basic documents as: "not only the absence of disease and infirmity but also the presence of physical, mental and social well-being." By introducing well-being as an objective in health care, a subjective element is introduced. Not only the symptom (health, functional or performance status) is registered, but also the way the symptom is perceived by the patient. For example in case of urinary incontinence the leakage of urine may cause irritation and itching of the skin in the genital area. This affects the physical well-being. The embarrassment caused by the possible smell as well as frequent visits to the toilet do affect social well-being, while the subsequent isolation affects the patient's mental well-being. The designing of questionnaires to assess the patient's well-being is the field of clinimetry. All questionnaires should contain (sub)scales with regard to physical, psychological, social and functional well-being (dimensions) and should be validated to ascertain that they are reliable and appropriate for the medical condition that is under study. The internal consistency (Crohnbach's alpha) measures the understanding ability of the questions, while the reproducibility is tested by the assessment of the inter-observer variation. The outcome of the questionnaire is then compared in two groups of patients with and without the medical condition under study (construct validity) and to a concurrent, validated questionnaire. Generic questionnaires such as the Short Form 36 (SF36) measure general well-being, while health-related quality-of-life (HR-QOL) instruments measure the quality-of-life related to a specific medical condition. The HR-QOL instruments are more suited to measure changes over time (responsiveness). The use of QOL-instruments has become more common in research as well as in daily practice. Generally, a generic questionnaire and a HR-QOL instrument are combined.

Because of the large and still increasing number of different pelvic floor QOL questionnaires available, comparison of outcome data between centers and populations is difficult. Furthermore, the availability of questionnaires in a broad range of languages is limited. In this context it should be realized that simple translation is not equal to validation. Current HR-QOL-validated questionnaires recommended in the field of pelvic floor dysfunction are the Urogenital Distress Inventory (UDI) (7), the Pelvic Floor Distress Inventory (PFDI) and the Pelvic Floor Impact Questionnaire (PFIQ) (18). These questionnaires address the urinary and faecal functioning as well as the distress caused by the mechanical symptoms of POP (pelvic heaviness and "bulging"). Currently, the trend is to reduce the number of questions to a "short form" that maintains its validity (19). If HR-QOL is measured before and after surgery, the questionnaire should be sufficiently responsive for changes in the condition. With the UDI and the Incontinence Impact Questionnaire IIQ7, a significant improvement of quality-of-life was found after incontinence or POP surgery (20). Ideally, we should reach a consensus in the forthcoming years about the most appropriate questionnaire to be used in pelvic floor dysfunction. Subsequently, this questionnaire should be made available in different languages through a well-designed validation process.

CLASSIFICATION OF POP

Before 1996 the classification of POP has been based on different scoring systems, depending on local rules and not based on a scientific validation. This resulted in poor reproducibility, which is particularly bothersome in clinical research, but also in a clinical setting where more than one doctor is examining the patient or where the patient will undergo several examinations during the follow-up after pelvic floor surgery. Lack of reproducibility could affect decision making in individual patients. Several scoring systems have been used, one of these being the halfway grading system (HWS), from grade 0 to 4, devised by Baden and Walker (8). This scoring system has been studied extensively, and has been widely accepted. Still more arbitrary scoring systems staged from incomplete to complete, mild to severe, from first degree to procidentia while using ill-defined landmarks such as the introitus instead of the hymen.

The criteria for an ideal classification, as defined by Baden and Walker (8), are:

- Easy to perform (or it will not be used);
- Easy to remember (or it will not be used correctly);
- Accurately defined (or it will be inconsistent);
- Adaptable to the needs of all—student, clinician, researcher and patient;
- Equally applicable at all six vaginal sites;
- Performed with the patient straining, to evaluate the defects at their worst;
- Assessed in relation to established, fixed landmarks along the vaginal canal;
- Graded for severity on a 0 to 4 basis to allow greater precision above the hymeneal level where most reparative procedures are performed; and
- Identified as the grading classification to immediately differentiate it from all other classifications.

Summarizing: the scoring system must weigh acceptability and practicability with the amount of reliable information. The system must be accepted by all uro-gynecologists to enable comparison between different centers and populations.

HISTORY OF POP CLASSIFICATION

In 1968, Baden and Walker (21) presented the "vaginal profile" because they felt that there was "an inability to communicate meaningful information about a common gynecologic problem." This scoring system was also known as the Original Grading Classification (OGC) (Table 2). This scoring system was not adopted by the profession, which was, at that time, attributed to several factors. The OGC required scoring all six sites from 0 to 4: urethra,

Table 2 Classification Systems and Characteristics

	OGC	HWS	POP-Q
Year of introduction	1968	1992	1996
All sites should be scored	X	–	X
Hymen reference point	X	X	X
Quantification (cm)	–	–	X
Halfway score (0–4)	X	X	–
Resulting in vaginal profile	X	–	X

Abbrevations: OGC, original grading classification; HWS, halfway grading system; POP-Q, Pelvic Organ Prolapse-Quantification.

bladder, cervix/cuff, pouch of Douglas, rectum and perineum. The scoring resulted in a number sequence (23,30,34). This was considered impractical. Another factor was the unusual method to score the culdo- (entero)-cele and the perineal descent, generating confusion. The final decision by the American College of Obstetrics and Gynecologists (ACOG) was that the OGC was, at that moment in time, complicated and laborious. As Baden and Walker later stated (8) "the gynecologists simply gave up." The ACOG recommended devising a more simple scoring system. In 1992, Baden and Walker presented their HWS (8). This classification required only the grading of the worst site or worst compartment, as desired by the examiner and as indicated by the patient's needs. The scoring of the culdocele was simplified according to the other sites. The scoring of the perineal descent was adapted (Table 3). Although the expectations of simplicity were met, the validation studies were scarce and inconsistent. In the presenting chapter of the HWS, a preliminary study of 25 patients was reported (8). The κ-value as a measure of inter-observer variation ranged from 0.70 to 1.0 for the different sites, while with respect to the anterior, apical and posterior compartment, the κ-values were 0.83, 0.78 and 0.85, respectively. This good reproducibility could not be confirmed in another

Table 3 Halfway Grading System[a] Devised by Baden and Walker with Respect to the Prolapse Sites 1–5[b]

Descend site 1–5	Grade	Perineal descent site 6
None	0	Normal
Halfway hymen	1	Halfway to sphincter
To hymen	2	To anal sphincter
Halfway past hymen	3	Involves anal sphincter
Maximum descent	4	Involves rectal mucosa

[a]An adapted scoring system for perineal descent (site 6).
[b]Urethra, bladder, uterine cervix or cuff, Douglas pouch, rectum.
Source: From Ref. 8.

study with κ's ranging from 0.27 to 0.50 (22). This has been the main argument to study the quantification of the assessment of prolapse.

At the same time a review appeared of 103 articles on pelvic floor surgery, it was found that only 61 authors used any grading systems at all and of the 61 articles that reported using a classification system only 10 utilized well-defined criteria (23). From the gynecological textbooks reviewed, one out of 15 revealed to have a well-defined classification system for POP. From this utter state of confusion came the most current and complete system for classifying POP, the POP-Q, notwithstanding the fact that it was remarkably similar to the formerly abandoned original grading system (OGC) (Table 2). In 1993, an international multidisciplinary committee comprising members of the ICS, the American Uro-Gynecologic Society and the Society of Gynecologic Surgeons drafted a standard document that has been adopted by the ICS in October 1995. In 1996, the POP-Q system was published by Bump (6).

THE POP-QUANTIFICATION

The POP-Q is characterized by six well-defined points on the vagina: two points in the anterior compartment, two points in the apical compartment and two points in the posterior compartment. These points (Aa, Ba, Ap, Bp, C and D) are shown in Figure 2.

Point Aa is located in the midline of the anterior vaginal wall 3 cm proximal to the external urethral meatus. Point Ba represents the most distal position of any part of the upper anterior vaginal wall from the vaginal cuff or anterior vaginal fornix to point Aa. Point C represents either the most distal edge of the cervix or the leading edge of the vaginal cuff (hysterectomy scar) after total hysterectomy. Point D is only described if the uterine cervix is present and represents the location of the posterior fornix (or Douglas pouch) where the sacrouterine ligaments are attached to the posterior side of the cervix. Point Bp represents the most distal position of any part of the upper posterior vaginal wall from the vaginal cuff or posterior vaginal fornix to point Ap. Point Ap is located in the midline of the posterior vaginal wall 3 cm proximal to the hymen. The hymen will be the fixed point of reference used throughout this system of quantitative prolapse description. The anatomic position of the six defined points for measurement should be centimeters above or proximal to the hymen (negative numbers) or centimeters below or distal to the hymen (positive numbers). By definition, the range of position of the points Ap and Aa relative to the hymen is −3 cm to +3 cm. In addition, the length of the perineal body, the genital hiatus and the vagina total vaginal length-TVL are measured. All the values can be documented in a grid and graphically depicted as a vaginal profile (Fig. 3). Finally an order can be assigned according to the most severe portion of the prolapse when the full extent of the descent has been

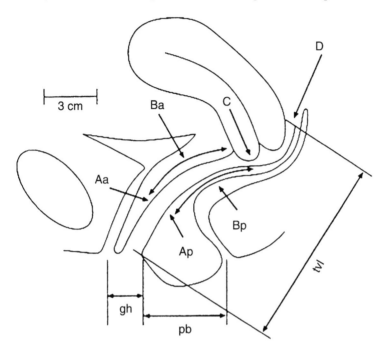

Figure 2 The different anatomical sites of pelvic organ prolapse (POP) with nine points used for POP quantification: points Aa, Ba, C, D, Bp, and Ap, genital hiatus (hg), perineal body (bp), and total vaginal length (TVL). *Source*: From Ref. 6.

demonstrated. Stage 0: no prolapse is demonstrated; Stage I: deepest part of the prolapse <-1 cm; Stage II: deepest part >-1 cm but $<+1$ cm; Stage III: deepest part $>+1$ cm, but protrudes no further than 2 cm less than the total vaginal length in centimeters; Stage IV: total eversion of the vagina, deepest part of prolapse $+$ TVL-2 cm.

    In a blinded study comprising 49 patients with POP or urinary incontinence, and comparing the POP-Q score with the HWS, both classifications had a good inter-observer agreement (κ's > 0.60 in all sites) (24). The inter-observer agreement of the POP-Q score was good for the stages (Stage 0: 0.79; Stage I: 0.85; Stage II: 0.79; Stage III: 0.82; Stage IV: 0.79) as well as for the individual sites. The POP-Q performed better (κ: 0.79) than the HWS (τ 0.68). In yet another comparative blinded study, a good correlation was found between both scoring systems (25). Hall reported good intra-observer agreement in 25 subjects with POP (26).

    To confirm that the POP-Q score really measures POP, a pelvic floor symptom score (five symptoms) was compared with the POP-Q score in patients who were seen for a routine gynecological visit (9). As the author reported earlier in this chapter, the number of positive responses increased

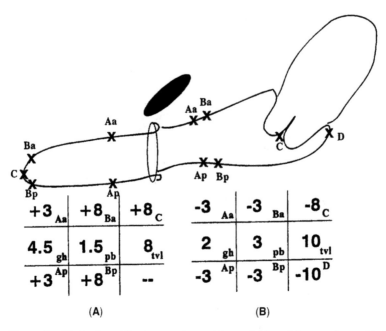

Figure 3 Vaginal profiles in a patient without POP and in a patient with Stage IV prolapse of the uterus.

according to POP-Q stage. In Stage III, more than two questions had a positive response compared to 0.86 questions in Stage II. In the same study population other factors that are associated with POP such as advancing age, increasing gravidity and parity, increasing number of vaginal births, delivery of a large birth weight infants, history of hysterectomy or POP surgery, were correlated to the POP-Q stage as well (27).

The scoring system is gradually accepted, at least by the members of the International Association of Uro-Gynecology (IUGA), 44% of its members have been known to report to use the system in daily practice (28). Some of the presumed shortcomings can be refuted easily. The learning curve is short. After instruction with a 17-min video on the POP-Q score 51 residents and students were able to interpret the examination findings up to 3 months (29). Having completed the learning curve, the POP-Q score takes 2 to 3 min. The examiner needs a Sims speculum, a bivalve speculum and a ruler or calibrated forceps. During the POP-Q score the patient is supposed to strain as much as possible and the examiner should describe the maximum protrusion. Sometimes it may be necessary that the patient stands while she is examined, in spite of the fact that there has been no statistically significant difference reported between the stage or any of the measured points in the dorsal lithotomic or standing examinations (30).

Not all the pelvic floor examination techniques have been incorporated in the POP-Q score and some will have to be performed additionally if appropriate: combined vaginal/rectal examination to detect enterocele, the strength of the pelvic floor muscles and the sphincter ani, the assessment of lateral anterior wall defects and the measurement of the perineal descent.

CONCLUDING REMARKS

Particularly in the case of intended prolapse surgery, the objective assessment of the severity of the pelvic floor problem is of utmost importance. This implies using validated techniques in classifying the stage of POP and the POP-Q, the latter qualification takes the subjective perception of health problems into account apart from the mere symptoms.

REFERENCES

1. Mant J, Painter R, Vessey M. Epidemiology of genital prolapse: observations from the Oxford Family Planning Association Study. Br J Obstet Gynaecol 1997; 104:579–85.
2. Olsen AL, Smith VJ, Bergstrom JO, Colling JC, Clark AL. Epidemiology of surgically managed pelvic organ prolapse and urinary incontinence. Obstet Gynecol 1997; 89:501–6.
3. Thom D. Variation in estimates of urinary incontinence prevalence in the community: effects of differences in definition, population characteristics, and study type. J Am Geriatr Soc 1998; 46:473–80.
4. Nelson R, Norton N, Cautley E, Furner S. Community-based prevalence of anal incontinence. JAMA 1995; 274:559–61.
5. DeLancey JO. Anatomy and biomechanics of genital prolapse. Clin Obstet Gynecol 1993; 36:897–909.
6. Bump RC, Mattiasson A, Bo K, et al. The standardization of terminology of female pelvic organ prolapse and pelvic floor dysfunction. Am J Obstet Gynecol 1996; 175:10–7.
7. van der Vaart CH, de Leeuw JR, Roovers JP, Heintz AP. Measuring health-related quality of life in women with uro-genital dysfunction: the uro-genital distress inventory and incontinence impact questionnaire revisited. Neurourol Urodyn 2003; 22:97–104.
8. Baden WF, Walker T. Fundamentals, symptoms, and Classification. In: Baden WF, Walker T, eds. Surgical repair of vaginal defects. Philadelphia: Lippincott Company; 1992. pp. 9–23.
9. Swift SE, Tate SB, Nicholas J. Correlation of symptoms with degree of pelvic organ support in a general population of women: what is pelvic organ prolapse? Am J Obstet Gynecol 2003; 189:372–77.
10. Ellerkmann RM, Cundiff GW, Melick CF, Nihira MA, Leffler K, Bent AE. Correlation of symptoms with location and severity of pelvic organ prolapse. Am J Obstet Gynecol 2001; 185:1332–7.
11. Mouritsen L, Larsen JP. Symptoms, bother and POPQ in women referred with pelvic organ prolapse. Int Urogynecol J Pelvic Floor Dysfunct 2003; 14:122–7.

12. Scientific Committee of the First International Consultation on incontinence. assessment and treatment of urinary incontinence. Lancet 2000; 355:2153–8.
13. Handa VL, Harvey L, Cundiff GW, Siddique SA, Kjerulff KH. Sexual function among women with urinary incontinence and pelvic organ prolapse. Am J Obstet Gynecol 2004; 191:751–6.
14. Weber AM, Walters MD, Piedmonte MR. Sexual function and vaginal anatomy in women before and after surgery for pelvic organ prolapse and urinary incontinence. Am J Obstet Gynecol 2000; 182:1610–5.
15. Petros PE. New ambulatory surgical methods using an anatomical classification of urinary dysfunction improve stress, urge and abnormal emptying. Int Urogynecol J Pelvic Floor Dysfunct 1997; 8:270–7.
16. Fialkow MF, Gardella C, Melville J, Lentz GM, Fenner DE. Posterior vaginal wall defects and their relation to measures of pelvic floor neuromuscular function and posterior compartment symptoms. Am J Obstet Gynecol 2002; 187:1443–8.
17. World Health Organisation (WHO). Handbook of basic documents. Geneva: 1952.
18. Barber MD, Kuchibhatla MN, Pieper CF, Bump RC. Psychometric evaluation of 2 comprehensive condition-specific quality of life instruments for women with pelvic floor disorders. Am J Obstet Gynecol 2001; 185:1388–95.
19. Avery K, Donovan J, Peters TJ, Shaw C, Gotoh M, Abrams P. ICIQ: a brief and robust measure for evaluating the symptoms and impact of urinary incontinence. Neurourol Urodyn 2004; 23:322–30.
20. FitzGerald MP, Kenton K, Shott S, Brubaker L. Responsiveness of quality of life measurements to change after reconstructive pelvic surgery. Am J Obstet Gynecol 2001; 185:20–4.
21. Baden WF, Walker T, Lindsey JH. The vaginal profile. Tex Med 1968; 64:56–73.
22. Geomini PMAJ, Mol BWJ, Bremer GL, Brolmann HAM. Inter-observer Reproducibility of the Halfway Grading System: A scoring system for assessment of pelvic organ prolapse. J Gynecol Surg 2000; 16:79–82.
23. Brubaker L, Norton P. Current clinical nomenclature for description of pelvic organ prolapse. J Pelvic Surg 1993; 2:257–9.
24. Kobak WH, Rosenberger K, Walters MD. Inter-observer variation in the assessment of pelvic organ prolapse. Int Urogynecol J Pelvic Floor Dysfunct 1996; 7:121–4.
25. Bland DR, Earle BB, Vitolins MZ, Burke G. Use of the pelvic organ prolapse staging system of the International Continence Society. American Urogynecologic Society, and Society of Gynecologic Surgeons in perimenopausal women. Am J Obstet Gynecol 1999; 181:1324–7 (discussion).
26. Hall AF, Theofrastous JP, Cundiff GW, et al. Interobserver and intra-observer reliability of the proposed International Continence Society, Society of Gynecologic Surgeons, and American Urogynecologic Society pelvic organ prolapse classification system. Am J Obstet Gynecol 1996; 175:1467–70 (discussion).
27. Swift SE. The distribution of pelvic organ support in a population of female subjects seen for routine gynecologic health care. Am J Obstet Gynecol 2000; 183:277–85.

28. Davila GW, Ghoniem GM, Kapoor DS, Contreras-Ortiz O. Pelvic floor dysfunction management practice patterns: a survey of members of the international urogynecological association. Int Urogynecol J Pelvic Floor Dysfunct 2002; 13:319–25.
29. Steele A, Mallipeddi P, Welgoss J, Soled S, Kohli N, Karram M. Teaching the pelvic organ prolapse quantization system. Am J Obstet Gynecol 1998; 179: 1458–63 (discussion).
30. Swift SE, Herring M. Comparison of pelvic organ prolapse in the dorsal lithotomy compared with the standing position. Obstet Gynecol 1998; 91: 961–94.

3

Cystodefecography

Danielle Hock

Department of Radiology, CHC Clinique St. Joseph, Liège, Belgium

INTRODUCTION

Colpocystodefecography (CCD) (1) is an easy and quick radiolopical procedure that provides the clinician with a complete morpho-dynamic study of
the female pelvis.

It may be performed with radiological equipment in common use—
provided there is a camera allowing the acquisition of dynamic sequences—
and is thus available at low cost to any department of radiology.

Since the study is performed in a sitting position (i.e., as close as
possible to physiological stress conditions), uses barium as the main contrast
agent, and allows full visualization of the different pelvic compartments, it
provides a complete demonstration not only of pelvic prolapses, but also of
the mechanism and causes of dyschezia.

METHOD

CCD may be considered as both a simplification of Béthoux and Bory's
colpocystogram (2) and a modification in the direction of a more dynamic
approach. It is a combination of voiding cystography (3) and defecography
(4) in patients whose vagina has previously been opacified by inserting a
barium paste.

Opacification Stage

Opacification is performed by a nurse or technician in an adjacent room
and takes 5 to 10 minutes. After urethral catheterization and repletion of

the bladder with 250 ml of Isopaque-cysto, the urethra is opacified by injection of 1 ml of thick sterile barium paste through the tip of a syringe inserted at the urethral meatus. The vagina is then filled with 50 ml of the same thick sterile barium paste, also injected through the tip of a syringe inserted deep in the vagina. Finally, the rectum is filled with approximately 300 cc of a solid mixture of dehydrated potato chips and liquid barium (Micropaque).

Radiological Study

This procedure is also performed by the nurse or technician and takes approximately 5 to 10 minutes and is both static and dynamic.

Static Study

The patient is first in a standing position, and two side views are taken: one at rest (Fig. 1A), the other during a Valsalva maneuver (Fig. 1B). The purpose of these two images is to study the bladder and detect factors predisposing to stress incontinence (measurement of urethro-trigonal angle and appreciation of the bladder neck efficiency). They also permit the observation of internal sphincter ani.

The patient is then seated on a special defecography stool-chair, and two other side views are taken: one at rest (Fig. 1C), the other during a strong squeezing effort (Fig. 1D). These are intended to demonstrate a possible descending perineum and to appreciate the tonicity of the pelvic floor muscles (the ano-rectal junction should rise significantly during the squeezing effort), and to evaluate the external sphincter ani.

Dynamic Study: A dynamic sequence at the rate of 2 frames/sec is recorded during micturition and defecation, and a final picture is taken after maximal rectum and bladder emptying, during another strong defecation strain (Figs. 2A–2D). This demonstrates the reciprocal influences of the pelvic organs and allows full visualization of both internal and external prolapses.

IMAGE INTERPRETATION

Normal appearances and descriptions of various anomalies for the bladder, vagina, uterus, pouch of Douglas and rectum are as follows.

Bladder

Normal position and appearance: The bladder neck and floor are at the level of the mid-section of the pubic bone, the bladder neck is closed and the urethro-trigonal angle is 90° (Fig. 1A).

Bladder neck insufficiency: The bladder neck is open at rest and/or during the Valsalva maneuver (Fig. 1B).

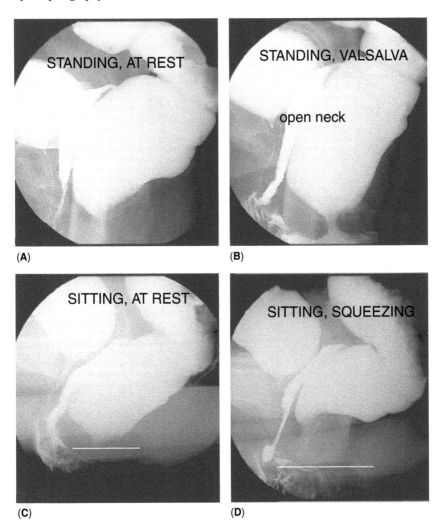

Figure 1   Static study. (**A**) Standing, at rest, aiming at the study of the bladder: there is no cystoptosis, the bladder neck is closed, and the utretho-trigonal angle is normal. (**B**) Standing, during a Valsalva maneuver (appreciation of bladder neck and internal sphincter ani efficiency). There is abnormal aperture of the bladder neck and of the anal canal, which betrays an insufficient internal sphincter ani. (**C**) Sitting, at rest, aiming at the recognition of a descending perineum, which is not present as the ano-rectal junction projects above the inferior aspect of the ischiatic bone (white line). (**D**) Sitting, during a strong squeezing effort, aiming at the appreciation of pelvic floor muscles tonicity (shown clearly in this figure, as the ano-rectal junction raises significantly above its position at rest, and as the ano-rectal angle closes in comparison to its value at rest), and at the appreciation of external sphincter ani (also effective as the anal canal is closed and lengthens normally).

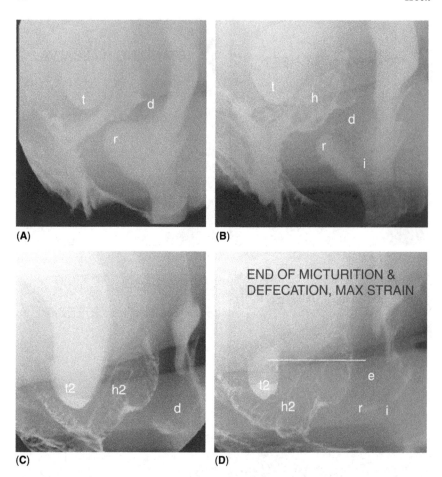

Figure 2   Dynamic study, micturition, and defecation are recorded at the rate of 2 images/sec. Dynamics of micturition and defecation (**A–C**). Final picture taken during a strong defecation strain (**D**) after maximal bladder and rectum emptying. *Bladder*: there is a trigonocele (*t*) as the trigone is below the level of the neck. It is graded II, as it reaches the level of the vulva. *Uterus*: the hysterocele (*h*) is seen as a mass encroaching progressively on the vaginal lumen and is graded II as it reaches the level of the vulva. *Pouch of Douglas:* at the beginning of defecation, the pouch of Douglas (*d*) is seen between the rectal anterior and vaginal posterior walls, which are still in contact in their lower parts (**A**), it then deepens progressively (**B, C**) and separates totally the rectum and the vagina, leading to the constitution of an enterocele (**D**). *Rectum*: there is a descending perineum [the anorectal junction is below the inferior margin of the ischiatic bone (white line)] and pelvic floor muscles are insufficient (the anorectal angle is totally open as it reaches 180°). An anterior intussusception (*l*) starts above the rectocele (*r*) (**B**) and slides into the upper portion of the anal canal, without hindering the rectocele evacuation, probably because of the positive squeezing effect exerted by the retrovaginal enterocele (*e*).

Cystoptosis: The neck and the trigone are below the level of the pubic bone mid-section.

Trigonocele: The trigone is below the level of the neck, which is in the correct position (Figs. 2A– 2C).

Sphincter hypertony: during micturition, the bladder contracts violently (irregular walls with possible diverticula), the bladder neck opens too widely, and the urethral distal portion appears too thin.

Vagina

Normal position and appearance: The vagina has a posterior-oblique direction and a virtual, empty lumen. The uterine neck is outlined in its upper portion (Figs. 1D).

Following cystopexy: The proximal part of the vagina and its distal third form an angle whose apex remains in close contact with the inferior aspect of the pubic bone during micturition and defecation strain (Figs. 3A and 3B).

Following sacral fixation: The full length of the vagina appears fixed and stretched, the same appearance being maintained during micturition and defecation strain (Figs. 3C and 3D).

Uterus

Normal position and appearance: the uterine cervix is seen as a mass encroaching on the apex or the upper third of the opacified vagina (Figs. 1A– 1D).

Hysterocele (uterine prolapse): the uterus is seen as a mass encroaching on half or more of the vaginal lumen, or descending to the level of the vulva (Figs. 2A– 2D).

Pouch of Douglas

Normal position and appearance: the pouch of Douglas is not visible as it is situated at the intersection of the vaginal apex, the uterine neck, and the anterior rectal wall (Fig. 4A).

Deep pouch of Douglas: the pouch of Douglas is seen as a mass determining a partial dissection between the anterior rectal and the posterior vaginal walls (Fig. 4B).

Retro-vaginal enterocele: the dissection of the anterior rectal and posterior vaginal walls is complete, and the Douglas pouch is seen as a mass reaching the vulva level (Fig. 5A).

Endo-vaginal enterocele: after hysterectomy, the Douglas pouch slides into the vaginal lumen, and is seen as a mass identical to a hysterocele (Fig. 5B).

Anterior enteric prolapse: after hysterectomy, the Douglas pouch may slide between the anterior vaginal wall and the bladder.

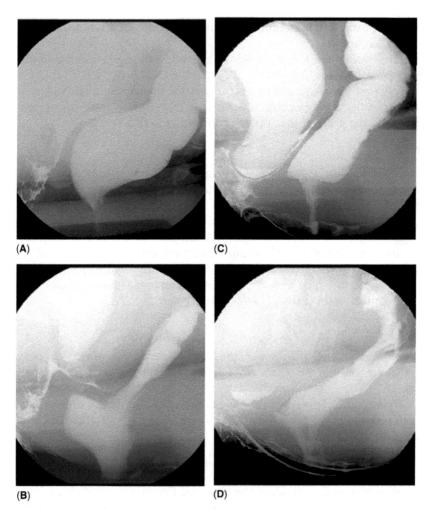

Figure 3 Vaginal appearance following surgery. Following cystopexy (**A,B**), the distal third and the proximal part of the vagina form an angle with the summit in close contact with the inferior aspect of the pubic bone. There is also a nonemptying rectocele. Following sacral fixation (**C,D**), the full length of the vagina appears stretched and fixed. There is a grade II-III trigonocele.

Rectum

1. *Normal position and appearance*: at rest, the rectum is nested in the sacral concavity, the anal canal is closed and situated above the level of the inferior aspect of the ischiatic bone (Figs. 1A– 1D).
2. *Descending perineum*: at rest, the anal canal is beyond the inferior aspect of the ischiatic bone (Fig. 5A).

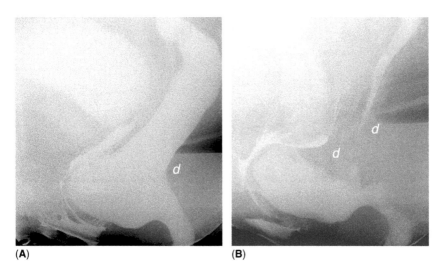

(A)   (B)

Figure 4 Pouch of Douglas in a case of hysterectomy. **(A)** The pouch of Douglas is not visible between the vaginal apex and the anterior rectal wall. Following defecation **(B)**, the pouch of Douglas (*d*) deepens and is seen as a mass between the upper part of the opacified vagina and the rectal anterior wall. Its descent is stopped by a non-emptying rectocele: should this symptomatic rectocele be resected without simultaneous resection of the pouch of Douglas, there is a risk of developing a post-operative enterocele.

3. *Rectal prolapse:* the rectum is more or less vertical and no longer follows the sacral concavity.
4. *Rectocele*: anterior bulging of the supra-anal part of the rectum, which only becomes pathologic when it is perceived by clinical evaluation and when the patient complains of incomplete rectal emptying (Figs. 4A and 4B).
5. *Intussusception*: invagination of the rectal wall, which may be anterior, posterior or circumferential and may lead to a solitary ulcer (Figs. 6A and 6B).
6. *Internal sphincter deficiency*: the anal canal is open at rest and/or opens during the Valsalva maneuver (Fig. 1B and Figs. 7A– 7C).
7. *External anal sphincter deficiency*: incomplete or nonexistent closure of the anal canal at maximal voluntary squeezing effort (Fig. 7D).
8. *External rectal prolapse*: in cases of anal sphincter deficiency, intussusception (often containing a large retro-vaginal enterocele) sliding through the enlarged anal canal and leading to rectal exteriorization (Figs. 8A and 8B)
9. *Pelvic floor muscles dyskinesia*: absence of relaxation or paradoxical contraction of pubo-rectalis and/or levator ani during defecation, often secondary or reflex to internal or external prolapses or to sphincter deficiencies (Figs. 9A and 9B).

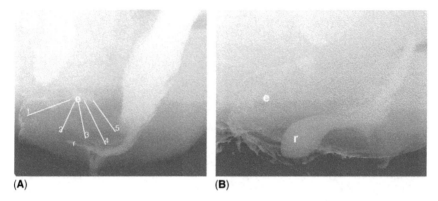

(A)   (B)

Figure 5 Retro- and endo-vaginal enteroceles in 2 cases of hysterectomy. **(A)** There is a large retro-vaginal enterocele (*e*), achieving a complete dissection between the vagina and the rectum: the mass reaches the level of the vulva. It squeezes the rectocele (*r*) and the lower portion of the rectum, hindering its proximal evacuation (negative squeezing effect). This patient also had cystopexy and sacral fixation: the proximal part of the vagina appears fixed and stretched and makes an angle with its distal part, the apex of which remains in close contact with the inferior aspect of the pubic bone. **(B)** The vagina is everted and contains an enterocele in its upper part, and a nonemptying rectocele in its lower part. This patient also had a cystopexy, which explains the intimate contact between the anterior vaginal wall and the inferior aspect of the pubic bone.

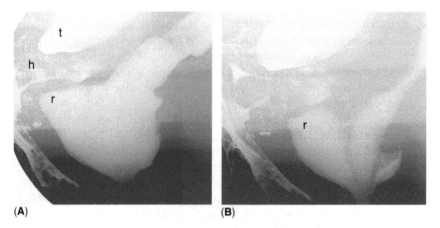

(A)   (B)

Figure 6 Intussusception. At the beginning of defecation **(A)**, there is a large rectocele (r). At this stage, the trigonocele (*t*) "sits" upon an endovaginal hysterocele (*h*). At the end of defecation **(B)**, there is a circumferential invagination of the rectal wall reaching the anal canal, secluding the rectocele and hindering its evacuation. The uterine neck cervix reaches the level of the vulva: grade III-IV hysterocele.

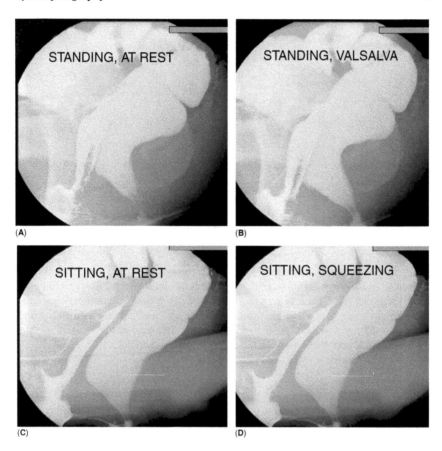

Figure 7 Sphincter ani. The anal canal remains open (**A–C**), which betrays an insufficient internal sphincter ani. During a strong squeezing effort (**D**), the anal canal does not close: there is also external sphincter ani insufficiency. The ano-rectal junction projects below the level of the inferior margin of the ischiatic bone (white line): descending perineum.

Reciprocal Influences

1. *Seated bladder descent*: the bladder floor is sustained by underlying prolapses which thus prevent its descent (a uterine prolapse, an endo-vaginal enterocele, an anterior enteric prolapse, a retro-vaginal enterocele or a rectocele) (Figs. 10A– 10D).
2. *Positive squeezing effect*: an enterocele may contribute, by extrinsic compression, to the good evacuation of the rectum or a rectocele (Figs. 11A and 11B).

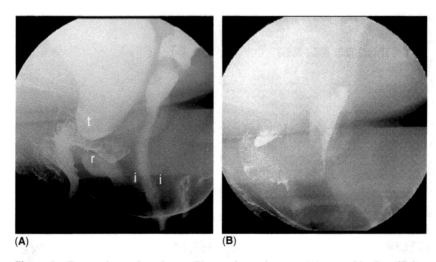

(A)   **(B)**

Figure 8 External rectal prolapse. The anal canal opens **(A)** too wide (insufficient sphincter) and there is an intra-anal circumferential intussusception (*i*) secluding a small rectocele (*r*). There is also a trigonocele (*t*) hiding an hysterocele (mass encroaching upon the proximal vaginal lumen). At the end of micturition and defecation **(B)**, the pouch of Douglas squeezes into the anterior part of the intussusception and there is a rectal external prolapse. There is a grade III-IV hysterocele sustaining a small "seated" trigonocele.

3. *Negative squeezing effect*: a retroflexed uterus (Fig. 10D), an enterocele, or a deep pouch of Douglas (Figs. 12A and 12B) may squeeze the rectum or the rectocele neck and impede their good evacuation.

ADVANTAGES OF CCD

In one single procedure, CCD collects all the information yielded by voiding cystography and defecography. On one hand it allows detection of cystoptosis, measurement of the urethro-trigonal angle, appreciation of the bladder neck competence, and study of the dynamics of micturition. On the other hand, it allows evaluation of levator ani, assessment of pubo-rectalis and anal sphincter tonicity, and performance of the dynamic study of defecation. The vagina is opacified by soaking its walls, thereby avoiding any luminal distension and permitting visualization of true deformation or prolapse.

By negative contrast, prolapses of the uterus and/or the pouch of Douglas are easily recognizable: uterine prolapse as well as post-hysterectomy enterocele manifest themselves by a mass encroaching on the vaginal wall.

During defecation, a progressive broadening of the space between the posterior vaginal and anterior rectal walls is typical of retrovaginal enterocele.

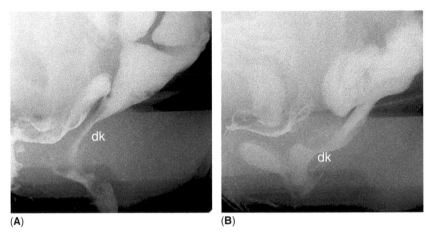

(A) (B)

Figure 9 Dyskinesia of pelvic floor muscles. The rectum rests posteriorly on the levator ani (**A**) so that the shape of posterior rectal wall reflects levator ani activity. The present concave form (*dk*) betrays levator ani paradoxical contraction at the end of defecation. Pubo-rectalis constitutes the upper part of sphincter ani (**B**). There is a posterior indentation (*dk*) in the upper portion of the ano-rectal junction, due to the absence of relaxation of the pubo-rectalis during defecation. The levator ani is in this case normally relaxed, as the posterior rectal wall appears convex. There is also a rectocele (*r*), secluded by a recto-intra-anal intussusception and a deep pouch of Douglas, seen as a mass between the vagina and the rectum.

The gravitational force acting in the sitting position and the Valsalva effort during defecation put the pelvic floor under severe strain and reveal its weak spots: CCD is the procedure of choice to detect prolapses and particularly enteroceles.

CCD demonstrates the reciprocal influences of pelvic components. For instance, a rectocele may sustain and mask a clinically silent trigonocele, a retrovaginal enterocele may compress the neck of a rectocele, and similarly, it may push the rectum downwards and cause its external prolapse through an insufficient anal sphincter. Thus, in addition to defecography *sensu stricto*, the visualization of the effects of neighboring structures on the rectal function completes the diagnosis.

COMPARISON OF CCD WITH CLINICAL EVALUATION

Based on a review of 300 examinations, Figure 13 compares the clinical evaluation and CCD in the diagnosis of the various types of pelvic prolapses. The radiological interpretation of the rectal parameters has to be distinguished from the others because it compares defecography directly with clinical evaluation. As it is now well demonstrated that a rectocele

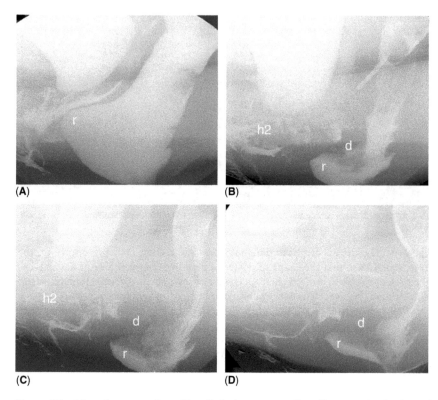

Figure 10 Negative squeezing effect linked to a retroflexed uterus. Beginning of defecation (**A**): there is a rectocele (*r*), a "seated" trigonocele, and a retroflexed uterus seen thanks to the IUD. Following micturition and defecation (**B–D**), uterine retroflexion is more marked, the uterus slides into the vagina with a subsequent grade II-III prolapse (*h2*), and its dome squeezes the lower portion of the rectum, hindering its proximal evacuation. Simultaneously, the pouch of Douglas pouch (*d*) insinuates enters between the uterus and the rectum and squeezes the rectocele neck. There is also a recto-intra-anal intussusception secluding the rectocele.

shown only by defecography may have no clinical relevance (5), Figure 13 takes only the non-emptying cases into account. Despite that restriction, an important discrepancy remains between the radiologically diagnosed rectoceles (255/300 = 75%) and the clinically diagnosed and radiologically confirmed lesions (70/300 = 23%).

This observation of a large number of radiologically diagnosed albeit clinically silent rectoceles is in agreement with recent work suggesting that the significance and prognostic value of defecography should be treated with caution. Radiological findings are indeed useful to strengthen clinical evaluation, but in the absence of subjective complaints they are insufficient to justify surgical correction.

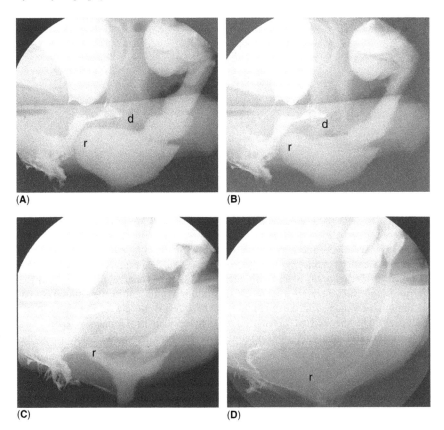

(A) (B)

(C) (D)

Figure 11 Positive squeezing effect linked to an enterocele in a patient who had hysterectomy and cystopexy. At the beginning of defecation **(A)**, there is a rectocele (*r*) and the pouch of Douglas (*d*) begins to slide between the vagina and the rectum. The vagina makes an angle, the summit apex of which is in close contact with the inferior margin of the pubic bone (cystopexy). Following rectum and bladder emptying **(B–D)**, the pouch of Douglas deepens progressively and dissects completely the recto-vaginal space, with the constitution of an enterocele. This enterocele squeezes progressively the rectocele, helping its total evacuation: a positive effect on the defecation.

With regard to other pelvic organs, there was good agreement between the clinical evaluation and CCD in 62 to 78 percent of cases. The degree of concordance decreases when all the pelvic prolapses occurring in the same patient are considered (Fig. 14). The false positive and, particularly, the numerous false negative diagnoses based on clinical grounds probably result from the conditions in which the clinical examination is performed.

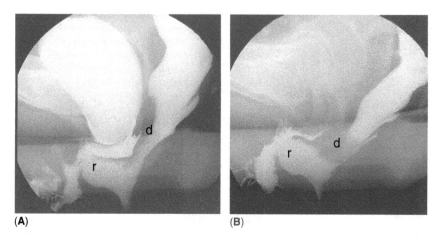

(A)   **(B)**

Figure 12 Negative squeezing effect linked to a deep pouch of Douglas in a patient who had hysterctomy and cystopexy. At the beginning of defecation (**A**), the pouch of Douglas (*d*) is normally comprised between the vaginal apex and the anterior rectal wall. There is a rectocele (r) and an angulation in the vaginal shape, the summit of which is in close contact to the inferior margin of the pubic bone (cystopexy). At the end of defecation (**B**), the pouch of Douglas deepens and squeezes the rectum's mid-section, hindering its proximal evacuation (negative squeezing effect).

Indeed, the topography of the pelvic organs, especially the site, size, and possible plurality of prolapses, is related to the local tonicity of the pelvic floor and to surgical history. It should be emphasized that the strain on the pelvic floor will always be weaker when the patient is lying on the examination bed than when defecating in a sitting position. Finally, clinical examination requires a vaginal palpation and/or insertion of a speculum. In both instances, prolapses will be partially pushed backwards. Even when the vagina is everted, inspection and palpation do not easily identify the cause of vaginal prolapse. Eighty-four percent of the enteroceles recognized by CCD are missed by clinical examination. Although seldom present at rest, the enterocele usually manifests itself during the Valsalva maneuver and defecation. In fact, the pouch of Douglas fills the space freed during rectal emptying. This explains not only the difficulty of establishing clinical diagnosis of enteroceles, but also their more frequent occurrence after significant pelvic surgery.

PELVIC SURGERY AND RISK OF ENTEROCELE

Spontaneous enteroceles, observed in 21 percent of the patients in the absence of any history of significant pelvic surgery, are linked neither to aging nor to multiparity.

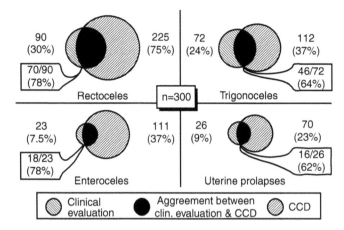

Figure 13 Comparison of clinical evaluation and Colpocystodefecography performances in diagnosing each of the pelvic prolapses.

Surgery of the pelvis increases the risk of enteroceles. Their incidence rises following a modification of organ volume (surgical cure of rectocele), or of position (cystopexy), and above all, following hysterectomy coupled or not with cystopexy and/or rectal surgery (Fig. 15).

CONCLUSION

CCD is a rapid and relatively easy radiological procedure that has proved to be a useful adjunct to clinical examination for the diagnosis of prolapses and particularly of the herniation of the pouch of Douglas hernia, i.e., enterocele.

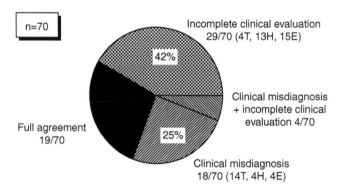

Figure 14 Comparison of clinical evaluation and Colpocystodefecography performances in diagnosing all of the prolapses of the same patient, in the 70 patients with a clinically diagnosed and radiologically confirmed rectocele. *Abbreviations*: E, enterocele; H, urine prolapse; T, trigonocele.

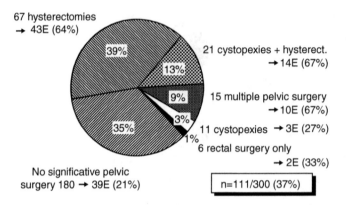

67 hysterectomies → 43E (64%)

21 cystopexies + hysterect. → 14E (67%)

15 multiple pelvic surgery → 10E (67%)

11 cystopexies → 3E (27%)

6 rectal surgery only → 2E (33%)

No significative pelvic surgery 180 → 39E (21%)

n=111/300 (37%)

Figure 15 Relationship between enterocele and pelvic history. *Abbreviation*: E, enterocele.

Moreover, CCD provides a complete morphologic and functional study of the female pelvis and demonstrates the interactions between pelvic organs, whether positive (supporting function or squeezing effect helping good evacuation) or negative (external lumen compression hindering proper emptying). This information is particularly helpful in deciding the type and extent of surgical intervention.

Indeed, in some instances, it will demonstrate the need to complete the surgical procedure by resection of the pouch of Douglas or by cysto- or hysteropexy, i.e., procedures intended to avoid potential postoperative complications such as prolapses and enteroceles.

REFERENCES

1. Hock D, Lombard R, Jehaes C, et al. Colpocystodefecography. Dis Colon Rectum 1993; 36:1015–21.
2. Zafiropulo M, Juras J, Boursier A, Scali P. Le colpocystogramme. In: Utilisation Actuelle des Explorations Instrumentales en Gynécologie (Sein exclu). Masson, 1983:374–84.
3. Olesen KP. Descent of the female urinary bladder. Dan Med Bull 1983; 30:66–84.
4. Mahieu P, Pringot J, Bodart P. Defecography I. Description of a new procedure and results in normal patients. Gastrointest Radiol 1984; 9:247–51.
5. Finlay IG. Symposium, proctography. Int J Colorectal Dis 1988; 3:67–89.

Part 2: The Anterior Segment

4

Urodynamic Investigations: Do They Make a Difference in the Outcome?

Jean Jacques Wyndaele

Department of Urology, Faculty of Medicine, University of Antwerp, Antwerp, Belgium

INTRODUCTION

Different factors related to the anatomy of the pelvic region contribute to the lower urinary tract (LUT) function in the female. For optimal continence, mechanisms related to the bladder, urethra, and pelvic floor have been identified (Table 1).

Proper diagnosis of any pathology in these factors is essential for the successful outcome of incontinence treatment. This chapter discusses the diagnostic techniques and their importance in deciding whether to perform continence surgery and for the outcome of such surgery.

DIAGNOSTIC TECHNIQUES FOR FEMALE INCONTINENCE

The diagnosis of female incontinence should be arrived at in the same manner as in most other medical conditions. It must commence with proper history taking, followed by clinical investigation. Urine analysis is necessary to exclude infection or other pathology of the urinary tract. Technical investigations may include imaging, rarely endoscopy or isotope investigation.

Homma (1) reviewed the literature before 2002 and included the review by Jensen et al. (2) on the role of history in the diagnosis of urinary incontinence. The conclusion was that when taking auxiliary information as age, surgical history, data from frequency–volume charts into account, urinary stress incontinence (USI) as the dominant symptom had a very high

Table 1   Factors Related to Female Continence

Upper urinary tract factors
   Ureters ending in bladder or proximal of urethral closure mechanisms

Lower urinary tract factors
   Bladder
   Sufficient capacity
   Filling at low pressure possible
   Detrusor normal active
   Bladder neck competent
   Normal micturition
   No post void residual
   No fistula

   Urethra
   Sufficient intrinsic resistance
   External sphincter integrity
   No obstruction anatomical or functional

   Pelvic floor
   Good support of bladder and urethra
   Good closing activity of urethra
   Proper relaxation during voiding

Note: No grading of importance of the different factors is given because this differs from case to case.

predictive value of genuine stress incontinence. This was also found by Maes-Wyndaele (3) in 100 incontinent women without neurological pathology: a good correlation between history and urodynamics was found in 80% of the women complaining of stress incontinence. However, complaints of urge or urge incontinence proved a poor predictor of detrusor over-activity (DOA). Nocturia, frequency, urgency or urge incontinence do not differ between stress and urge incontinence (4). The low predictive value of symptoms was even more evident in the geriatric population due to impaired cognitive ability and coexisting diseases (5).

   Homma also reminds us that there is a strong discrepancy between symptoms and urodynamic findings. Urodynamic testing is not always able to reproduce the symptoms. Symptoms and urodynamics often assess different aspects of the incontinence problem and therefore may have an adjunctive role in the overall diagnosis. However, this does not make urodynamics less valuable nor does it make history taking superfluous.

   One important aspect of the examination is the physician's observation of leakage on straining or coughing. This is a clear sign that USI is present, if the test is done in good conditions: sufficient bladder filling, development of high enough intra-abdominal pressure, leakage stops when coughing stops and urine does not continue to run out (what is suggestive for cough-induced DOA). In a large study group, Dwyer (6) found that where the sign of USI could be demonstrated, 91% had the actual diagnosis of USI. However, only 53% had USI alone. The other 38% had mixed USI and DOA, USI with hypersensitive bladder, or USI with voiding difficulties. The author concludes that the sign of USI, when present, permits to treat patients conservatively. But he does not find the sign of USI to be strong enough evidence on which to perform surgery, as 47% have another urodynamic diagnosis.

Urodynamic tests are the most specific tests for evaluating the LUT function. A short review of some of the commonly used tests follows.

URODYNAMIC TESTING

Urodynamic investigations have become an integral part of daily urological practice. The need for objectivation of LUT functions or dysfunctions, and the knowledge that this can improve diagnosis and treatment has helped to overcome the critical antipathy which has kept resistance against urodynamics for so long. The ever-improving knowledge about muscular, neurological and humoral factors involved in the continence–micturition cycle has helped to better understand how urodynamic function is best studied.

The last 10 years has seen an important evolution in the urodynamic equipment available on the market and this evolution continues towards less invasive, more patient-friendly and better focused on what one needs to measure.

Computerized systems created very sophisticated mathematical parameters; however, their clinical value has not always been submitted to in-depth evaluation. Long lists of numeric data are generated automatically but these can be misleading, they even can be wrong. Investigators should be aware of this. Urodynamic investigation is not a science in its own right. It is a diagnostic tool which offers several diagnostic possibilities that need to be correctly positioned in a complete diagnostic workout. Interpretation of the tests needs to be done individually, critically and should also rule out system- and technique-related mistakes. If these rules are followed, experience and scientific-based criticism will permit urodynamics to offer help in many clinical controversies.

The International Continence Society has done a tremendous work by publishing, on regular basis, reports on standardization of techniques and their interpretation, offering a solid base for investigation performance and interpretation (7,8). The general principles of urodynamic investigation are:

- to measure functional parameters related to the referring systems;
- to identify the parts of the LUT that are involved in the problem;

- to look for complementary data of importance for the therapeutic decision making;
- to try and explain why a treatment based on a tentative diagnosis has been unsuccessful.

The investigator will start from the symptoms, will design test in order to try and reproduce these symptoms during the test and in so doing find a functional explanation for these symptoms. This is an approach that opens the way to selective treatment.

Uroflow

This is the single most important test in clinical urodynamics. Uroflow measurement is generally obtained by voiding into a receptacle that converts changes in weight or momentum into an electrical signal that can be graphically displayed on a strip chart recorder. This time/volume recording can be used to calculate several parameters.

Urination is usually a private undertaking especially in women. Psychic factors can influence the quality of urination. The major challenge when planning an uroflow study is to provide a setting which does not make the study misrepresentative of the patient's normal experience. Several suggestions in methodology will prove useful (9):

- put the receptacle in a bathroom facility where the patient can be alone;
- avoid the need for the patient to turn on the machine herself when she is ready to void;
- let the patient urinate in her normal position (mostly sitting);
- instruct her to present herself with a "comfortable" full bladder, while avoiding bladder overfilling;
- ensure that she is not disturbed during voiding;
- instruct the patient beforehand about the purpose of the test and the technique used;
- inquire, after the test, if she considered the voiding process normal, in other words if it represented her usual voiding pattern;
- avoid, prior catheterization and thus pain and discomfort; although catheterization does not seem not to influence greatly the outcome of the flow.

Proper interpretation often requires more than one micturition. This can be achieved by asking the patient to drink beforehand but she should not change her voiding/drinking habit to prevent her to retain more urine than she is used to.

Parameters most frequently used are presented in Fig. 1. The relationship between flow rate and volume voided is well known. Below 150 or 200 ml voided, the curve would be considered less reliable. Evaluation of a post-mictional residual volume can be done by ultrasonography or catheterization.

The uroflow meter should be regularly controlled and kept clean. While the overall shape of the curve has some importance, there are limits to what can be deducted from it; this is especially true for uroflowmetry in incontinent women. It is widely assumed that normal micturition is reflected in a normal flow pattern (8). This would also mean that a normal flow curve would correspond to normal voiding and would permit to exclude voiding difficulties (10,11). However, Pauwels et al. (12) investigated the clinical meaning of a normal flow pattern in four different groups: stress incontinent women, women with bladder over-activity, healthy middle-aged volunteers and healthy students. It became evident that women who strained to void, a major component of dysfunctional voiding problems, produced a bell-shaped flow curve in, respectively, 46, 60, 70 and 100%. This study makes it clear that a "normal, bell-shaped" flow curve does not exclude voiding dysfunction in women.

Cystometry

Cystometry is defined as the recording of changes in intravesical pressure during bladder filling and micturition. The technique is useful to evaluate detrusor function (sensation, vesicosphincteric reflex, pressure/volume response, involuntary detrusor contraction), DOA, voluntary reflex contractions at capacity, and the patient's ability to suppress detrusor contractions voluntarily.

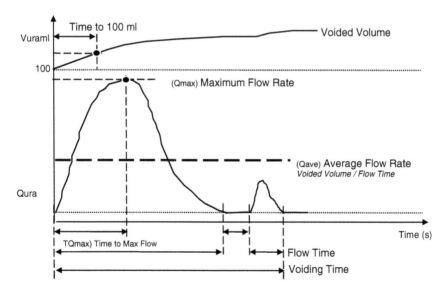

Figure 1 Flow curve and parameters for the most part automatically generated by the new type-flow meters.

In order to find a cystometric correlate for symptoms which occur during the filling-storage cycle, it is necessary to reproduce these symptoms during the study.

Methodological recommendations have also been developed for cystometry:

- Appraise the patient beforehand about the test and that she will be catheterized. Most often the catheter is inserted transurethrally. Any lubricant used for catheterization should be free of an anesthetic compound not to influence the outcome. Although the caliber of the catheter does not significantly affect the results of cystometry, if simultaneous flow rates are to be determined the catheter should not be larger than 10 French.
- Fluid-filled catheters linked to external transducers or micro-tip transducers can be used. There are methods for the zeroing of both.
- Calibration of the recording equipment must be precise.
- Pressure lines or transducers must be positioned correctly.
- It is essential to comply with proper standardized techniques to avoid artifacts.
- The physician should be present for on-the-spot interpretation and conclusion.
- An intra-abdominal line is needed. For this purpose a catheter is usually introduced into the rectum or less frequently into the vagina. The catheter must be positioned deep enough (10 cm intra-rectal) to obtain a reliable measurement of the intra-abdominal pressure. Some patients void with abdominal straining alone or strain to augment outflow during detrusor contraction. Some are anxious or restless and can induce brisk pressure rise by moving, coughing, and so on. Only if an abdominal pressure line is available, can the relative importance of these parameters be appreciated. It is useful to all pressure changes even if modern equipment shows rise in detrusor pressure (vesical pressure minus abdominal pressure automatically subtracted). Pure abdominal pressure variations can change detrusor pressure outcome themselves without any vesical activity.
- Water or aqueous radio-contrast solutions are the filling media of choice. The solution should be at least at room temperature or preferably at body temperature.
- Before filling starts, residual urine may be evacuated and measured. But one should realize that the removal of a large volume of residual urine may alter detrusor function.
- The patient should be awake and cooperative in order to yield maximum information.
- Drugs that affect bladder function should not be taken or should have been stopped if possible. If it is not possible to stop them, the investigator should account for their possible influence.

- The patient should preferably be in the position in which she experiences most of the symptoms.
- Filling can be done at infusion rate up to 20% of bladder capacity.
- Here again the purpose of the examination should be reiterated to the patient. She should be instructed to report sensations she experiences during filling and should be asked not to start voiding before warning the investigator.
- During filling the patient is periodically asked to cough and strain to check if the pressure lines are working correctly, to evaluate USI, and to provoke DOA. One must appreciate that the way coughing is done can greatly influence the eventual leaking of urine.

Many parameters can be controlled during filling of the bladder: bladder capacity, compliance and DOA (Fig. 2). The evaluation of the filling sensation is important as filling sensations guide for a major part of everyone's daily bladder control.

When the patient has a strong desire to void the pressure/flow study can start. The simultaneous measurement of intra-vesical pressure and flow during micturition is at present the best method of analyzing voiding function quantitatively. Direct inspection of the pressure and flow data is useful to get a first impression and is needed to exclude artifacts. DOA during micturition is as important as urethral external sphincter and bladder neck activity. Computerized quantifications of data are available and several

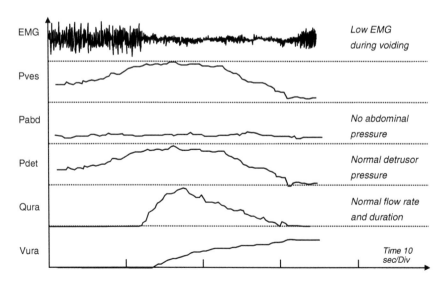

Figure 2   Curves of normal pressure/flow part of cystometry.

methods have been developed for the analysis of pressure/flow plots. They are used mostly for outflow problems.

The evaluation of urethral and bladder neck function can be done with urethral sphincter electromyography, continuous urethral pressure measurement, and videocystometry (Fig. 3).

Urethral Pressure Profile

Urethral pressure profile (UPP) is a graphic recording of the pressure within the urethra at each point along its length. Many factors influence urethral pressure: smooth muscle activity, blood flow through the urethral arteries and veins, fibro elastic tension of the wall, the mucosal folds, and striated muscle activity of the external sphincter and the pelvic floor. UPP recording is the result of all these. Techniques have been standardized.

The diagnostic value of a static UPP is not certain. It can be useful for the evaluation of sphincter-related incontinence, sphincterotomy, local treatment of sphincter dysfunctions as injection of local anesthetics, drug activity on urethral resistance, and so on.

Stress UPP is done with two pressure sensors, one in the bladder and one in the urethra (9). Another way to evaluate urethral resistance is with Valsalva leakpoint pressure (VLPP). The urodynamic parameters that need to be standardized for measurement of VLPP include urethral catheter size,

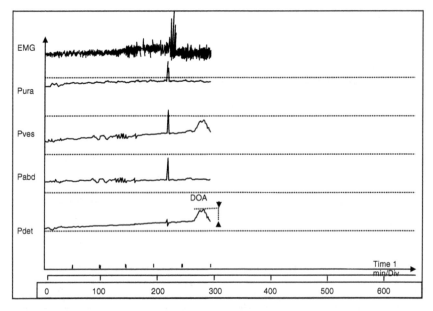

Figure 3   Filling cystometry with detrusor overactivity (DOA) on P_{ves} and P_{det} curve with electromyography increase.

zeroing of the transducer, position of the patient, bladder volume, type of stress, and timing of measurement (13).

The ICS standardization report on urethral pressure measurements was published in 2002 (14). It concluded that, at present, the clinical utility of urethral pressure measurement is unclear. There is no urethral pressure measurement that:

- discriminates urethral incompetence from other disorders;
- provides a measure of the severity of the condition;
- provides a reliable indicator of surgical success; and
- returns to normal after successful intervention.

Thus, urethral pressure measurement remains first and foremost a research tool.

CORRELATION BETWEEN SYMPTOM SEVERITY AND URODYNAMIC DATA

USI is caused by a deficiency of the dynamic urethral resistance. This incompetence of the urethral closure may be related to low maximum urethral closure pressure, low pressure transmission ratio, and/or low VLPP (15). In the literature the correlation between these measurements of urethral function and the presence or severity of USI varies greatly (1).

In DOA and urge incontinence the correlation between severity of urgency and amplitude or duration of DOA has not been demonstrated. Moreover, DOA has been described in healthy volunteers (16). So it would seem that the presence or severity of incontinence is not directly reflected in poor urodynamic functioning.

Urodynamic Parameters Related to the Outcome of Incontinence Surgery

The description of the techniques makes it evident that different urodynamic parameters relate to several incontinence-related factors listed in Table 1. The important factors for the bladder are: bladder capacity, bladder wall compliance, and detrusor activity during bladder filling and during voiding. The important factors for the outlet are: bladder neck competence, passive urethral resistance, and the urethral activity.

Detrusor Overactivity

DOA is an important outcome factor. In a meta-analysis of 48 studies, Hampel et al. (17) found a prevalence of incontinence in a mean of 23.6% of women; of these 51% were urge incontinence. The overall prevalence of overactive bladder with incontinence has been reported to be between 6% and 13% of the general population. The mean rate of combined stress incontinence and urge incontinence (mixed incontinence) has been reported as 29% of women living in the community (18). As mentioned earlier, history is a poor predictor of DOA. It has become clear that DOA leads to less satisfactory surgical outcome in cases of mixed incontinence, especially when it generates high vesical pressures. The incidence of postoperative urgency or urge incontinence is consistently higher if patients had symptoms beforehand (19). But in a proportion of patients, the symptoms will resolve (20).

Postoperative de novo DOA is another difficult problem. This may be a consequence of obstruction induced by surgery, of unrecognized over-activity that manifests itself postoperatively or of both (21,22). Its prevalence, after incontinence surgery, is between 10% and 20%. The prevalence is higher after sling than after Burch colposuspension (23). There is no urodynamic finding that is predictive of the development of de novo DOA or the persistence of previous DOA after surgery. If urgency and urge incontinence develop de novo, or remain after surgery, the satisfaction of the patient with the surgery is frequently compromised despite cure of the stress incontinence (24).

Detrusor Voiding Function

Permictional straining is common in women (25). Straining has been shown to be deleterious to the pelvic floor, as it may cause muscular and neurological lesions (26). The rate of success after incontinence surgery has been shown to be inferior with the use of slings (27). Others reported that voiding with valsalva and without proper detrusor contraction increases the risk of prolonged postoperative catheterization (28). Such voiding difficulties after incontinence surgery have been described in 32% of cases (29).

Uroflowmetry has been shown to be unreliable for the diagnosis of permictional straining (12). Urodynamic low peak flow rate and detrusor under-activity have been shown to be associated with post-surgery voiding difficulties (30,31). Measuring the isovolumetric contraction pressure or pressure/flow studies have not been highly predictive for postoperative voiding problems (32,33).

The measurement of isovolumetric contraction and pressure/flow studies aim at measuring the detrusor contractile function: But studies have shown that these measurements do not predict the voiding problems that can occur after incontinence surgery.

Intrinsic Sphincter Deficiency

The choice of surgical technique may be different if intrinsic sphincter deficiency (ISD) is diagnosed. An increase of urethral resistance will be searched for ISD cannot be diagnosed from symptoms and signs alone (34). Urodynamic techniques that indicate ISD are the measurement of maximal urethral closure pressure and leak point pressure. Bump et al. (35) compared three measurement techniques proposed to diagnose ISD: maximum urethral closure pressure (MUCP), VLPP and straining urethral axis. They found that only low closure and leak point pressures had significant associations with the severity of the incontinence. They rightly conclude that ISD should be diagnosed by a composite of historic, urodynamic, anatomic and clinical severity criteria. They propose the inclusion of a MUCP of ≤ 20, a VLPP of ≤ 50 and a stress urethral axis of ≤ 20 in this composite.

A correlation with external criteria (history, physical examination, anatomic findings and so on) would seem to be more evident for VLPP than for MUCP. Symptom severity correlates to some extent with VLPP but not with MUCP (36,37). A positive supine stress test with empty bladder or bladder filled to 200 ml is predictive for low VLPP but not for low MUCP (38,39).

The most important is a possible prediction of surgical outcome. If MUCP or VLPP are low then success rates with different surgeries are lower (40,41). However, studies have shown that a low MUCP is not a reliable predictor of surgical failure (42). ISD is a risk factor for persistent incontinence but sling surgery or urethropexy with further elevation of the urethra produce a high rate for continence associated with hypermobility, ISD or both. The discrimination of ISD by urodynamics may therefore perhaps become less critical in future. More studies are needed to make strong conclusions possible.

Limitations and Values of Urodynamic Tests

There are several shortcomings in the actual urodynamic tests:

- With urodynamic tests, the diagnosis can be missed altogether in a mean 9% of cases (3–25%) (2).
- Urodynamics can demonstrate data not related to the problem.
- The prevalence of DOA in a normal population has previously been noted.
- Symptoms do not relate well with urodynamics.
- Urodynamics are invasive.

On the other hand if one wants to investigate the different continence mechanisms by measuring the pressures and the resistance, urodynamic tests are the most specific and direct way to do this.

Surgery is invasive, even if "minimally invasive" techniques are used. The goal of surgery is to cure the patient. Diokno et al. (43) determined the prevalence of continence surgery and the outcome as reported by the patients in 24.581 women. Almost 4% had undergone continence surgery. The proportion of women initially satisfied with the results of surgery decreased from 67% to 45% who reported current satisfaction after a follow-up period of five years or longer. The continence rates were lower than most published figures, though some women reported satisfaction with surgery even when they did not achieve continence.

Do urodynamics help to improve the surgical outcome of incontinence surgery? Glazener and Lapitan (44) carried out a review for Cochrane Library in 2002–2003; they found only two studies that were acceptable for inclusion in the review which did not permit any conclusions to be reached. If urodynamic tests are not worthwhile to perform, what are the reasons? Theoretically several scenarios are possible: Is differentiation between symptomatic patients not possible because they all have the same pathology? Is the way urodynamics are performed mostly unreliable? Are the wrong tests chosen? Can't urodynamics predict outcome because wrong treatments are given? Some answers are clear: symptoms do not rely on the same pathology in all patients. Urodynamic tests need skill, knowledge and expertise and it is likely that not infrequently tests are done in an unreliable way or are interpreted wrongly.

As stated before, urodynamic tests are just one of several investigative methods and they should not stand alone. If a patient presents with urinary incontinence it is important to make a proper diagnosis as a result of the clinical assessment; in many cases sophisticated urodynamic tests are not necessary. A general assessment, frequency/volume chart, physical examination and proper stress tests will provide the physician with substantial information towards the diagnosis. If urinary tract infection is excluded and residual urine is absent, a presumptive diagnosis of stress, urge or mixed incontinence can be made and the patient started on conservative treatments such as pelvic floor physiotherapy, bladder training, life style adaptations and appropriate medications. However, it remains unclear if these data are sufficient to decide on undertaking surgery. One may argue that a patient with USI and no history of other symptoms or signs, corroborated with a complete diagnostic workout will have no strong need for urodynamic testing. However, there can be little doubt that urodynamic testing is necessary in patients who do not respond to conservative treatment or those who present with a more complex form of USI.

We must emphasize that, when performed or evaluated incorrectly, urodynamic tests provide no useful information. We must also emphasize that despite properly performed urodynamics, poorly selected or poorly performed incontinence surgery will yield bad results.

REFERENCES

1. Homma Y. The clinical significance of the urodynamic investigation in incontinence. BJU Int 2002; 90:489–97.
2. Jensen JK, Nielsen FR Jr, Ostergard DR. The role of patient history in the diagnosis of urinary incontinence. Obstet Gynecol 1994; 83:904–10.

3. Maes D, Wyndaele JJ. Correlation between history and urodynamics in neurologically normal incontinent women. Eur Urol 1988; 14:377–80.
4. Amundsen C, Lau M, English SF, McGuire EJ. Do urinary symptoms correlate with urodynamic findings? J Urol 1999; 161:1871–4.
5. Kirschner-Hermanns R, Scherr PA, Branch LG, Wetle T, Resnick NM. Accuracy of survey questions for geriatric urinary incontinence. J Urol 1998; 159:1903–8.
6. Dwyer PL. Differentiating urinary stress incontinence from urge urinary incontinence. Int J Gynec Obstet 2004; 86(Suppl. 1):S17–24.
7. Abrams P, Cardozo L, Fall M, Griffiths D, Rosier P, Ulmsten U, van Kerrebroeck P, Victor A, Wein A. The Standardisation of Terminology of Lower Urinary Tract Function: report from the Standardisation Sub-committee of the International Continence Society. Neurourol Urodyn 2002; 21:167–78.
8. Schäfer W, Abrams P, Liao L, Mattiasson A, Pesce F, Spanberg A, Sterling AM, Zinner NR, van Kerrebroeck P. Good urodynamic practices: uroflow-metry, filling cystometry, and pressure-flow studies. Neurourol Urodynam 2002; 21:261–74.
9. Wyndaele JJ. Methods for urodynamic investigation. Eur Urol 1998; 33:4–7.
10. Haylen BT, Parys BT, Anyaegbunam WI, Ashby D, West CR. Urine flow rates in male and female urodynamic patients compared with the liverpool nomograms. Br J Urol 1990; 65:483–7.
11. Jorgensen JB, Colstrup H, Frimodt-Moller C. Uroflow in women: an overview and suggestions for the future. Int Urogynecol J 1998; 9:33–6.
12. Pauwels L, De Wachter S, Wyndaele JJ. A normal flow pattern in women does not exclude voiding pathology. Int Urogynecol J Pelvic Floor Dysfunct 2005; 16:104–8.
13. Daneshgari F. Valsalva leak point pressure: steps toward standardization. Curr Urol Rep 2001; 2:388–91.
14. Lose G, Griffiths D, Hosker G, Kulseng-Hanssen S, Perucchini D, Schafer W, Thind P, Versi E. The standardisation of urethral pressure measurement. Neurourol Urodyn 2002; 21:258–60.
15. Khullar V, Cardozo L. The urethra (UPP, MUPP, instability, LPP). Eur Urol 1998; 34:20–2.
16. Wyndaele JJ. Normality in urodynamics studied in healthy adults. J Urol 1999; 161:899–902.
17. Hampel C, Wienhold D, Benken N, Eggersmann C, Thuroff JW. Definition of overactive bladder and epidemiology of urinary incontinence. Urology 1997; 50 (Suppl. 6):4–14.
18. Hunskaar S, Burgio K, Diokno AC, Herzog AR, Hjalmas K, Lapitan MC. Epidemiology and natural history of urinary incontinence. In: Abrams P, Cardozo L, Khoury S, Wein A (eds), Incontinence. Plymouth: Health Publications; 2002, p. 179.
19. Chaikin DC, Rosenthal J, Blaivas JG. Pubovaginal fascial sling for all types of stress incontinence: long-term analysis. J Urol 1998; 160:1312–6.
20. McGuire EJ, Savastano JA. Stress incontinence and detrsuor instability/urge incontinence. Neurourol Urodyn 1985; 4:313–6.

21. Bump RC, Copeland WE Jr, Hurt WG, Fantl JA. Dynamic urethral pressure/ profilometry pressure transmission ratio determinations in stress-incontinent and stress-continent subjects. Am J Obstet Gynecol 1988; 159:749–55.

22. Groutz A, Blaivas JG, Hyman MJ, Chaikin DC. Pubovaginal sling surgery for simple urinary stress incontinence: analysis by an outcome score. J Urol 2001; 165:1597–1600.

23. Griffiths D. Clinical aspects of detrusor instability and the value of urodynamics: a review of the evidence. Eur Urol 1998; 34:13–5.

24. Litwiller SE, Nelson RS, Fone PD, Kim KB, Stone AR. Vaginal wall sling: long-term outcome analysis of factors contributing to patients satisfaction and surgical success. J Urol 1997; 157:1279–82.

25. Karram MM, Partoll L, Bilota V, Angel O. Factors affecting detrusor contraction strength during voiding in women. Obstet Gynecol 1997; 90:723–6.

26. Marinkovic SP, Stanton SL. Incontinence and voiding difficulties associated with prolapse. J Urol 2004; 171:1021–8.

27. Iglesia CB, Shott S, Fenner DE, Brubaker L. Effect of preoperative voiding mechanism on success rate of autologous rectus fascia suburethral sling procedure. Obstet Gynecol 1998; 91:577–81.

28. Bhatia NN, Bergman A. Urodynamic predictability of voiding following incontinence surgery. Obstet Gynecol 1984; 63:85–91.

29. Jarvis GJ. Surgery for genuine stress incontinence. Br J Obstet Gynaecol 1994; 101:371–4.

30. Lose G, Jorgensen L, Mortensen SO, Molsted-Pedersen L, Kristensen JK. Voiding difficulties after colposuspension. Obstet Gynecol 1987; 69:33–8.

31. McLellan MT, Melock CF, Bent AE. Clinical and urodynamic predictors of delayed voiding after fascia lata suburethral sling. Obstet Gynecol 1998; 92: 608–12.

32. Norton P, Stanton SL. Isovolumetric detrusor tests-a predictor of post-operative voiding difficulties. Neurourol Urodyn 1988; 7:287–8.

33. Heit M, Vogt V, Brubaker L. An alternative statistical approach for predicting prolonged catheterization after Burch colpo suspension during reconstructive pelvic surgery. Int Urogynecol J Pelvic Floor Dysfunct 1997; 8:203–8.

34. McGuire EJ, Fitzpatrick CC, Wan J, Bloom D, Sanvordenker J, Ritchey M, Gormley EA. Clinical assessment of urethral sphincter function. J Urol 1993; 150:1452–4.

35. Bump RC, Coates KW, Cundiff GW, Harris RL, Weidner AC. Diagnosing intrinsic sphincteric deficiency: comparing urethral closure pressure, urethral axis, and Valsalva leak point pressures. Am J Obstet Gynecol 1997; 177: 303–10.

36. Cummings JM, Bouliier JA, Parra RO, Wozniak-Petrofsky J. Leak point pressures in women with urinary stress incontinence. J Urol 1997; 157:818–20.

37. Horbach NS, Ostergard DR. Predicting intrinsic urethral sphincter dysfunction in women with urinary stress incontinence. Obstet Gynecol 1994; 84:188–92.

38. Hsu TH, Rackley RR, Appell RA. The supine stress test: a simple method to detect intrinsic urethral sphincter dysfunction. J Urol 1999; 162:460–3.

39. McLellan MT, Bent AE. Supine empty stress test as a predictor of low Valsalva leak point pressure. Neurourol Urodyn 1998; 17:121–7.

40. Koonings PP, Bergman A, Ballard CA. Low urethral pressure and urinary stress incontinence in women: risk factor for failed retropubic surgical procedure. Urology 1990; 36:245–8.
41. Bowen LW, Sand PK, Ostergard DR, Frantl CE. Unsuccessful Burch retropubic urethropexy: a case-controlled study. Am J Obstet Gynecol 1989; 160:452–8.
42. Richardson DA, Ramahi A, Chals E. Surgical management of stress incontinence in patients with low urethral pressure. Gynecol Obstet Invest 1991; 31:106–9.
43. Diokno AC, Burgio K, Fultz NH, Kinchen KS, Obenchain R, Bump RC. Prevalence and outcomes of continence surgery in community dwelling women. J Urol 2003; 170:507–11.
44. Glazener CM, Lapitan MC. Urodynamic investigations for management of urinary incontinence in adults. Cochrane Database Syst Rev 2002; 3:CD003195.

5

Endoscopic Treatment: The Burch Procedure

John R. Miklos

Atlanta UroGynecology Associates, Alpharetta, Georgia, U.S.A.

Genuine urinary stress incontinence (GUSI) is defined by the International Continence Society (ICS) as the involuntary loss of urine coincident with increased intra-abdominal pressure in the absence of a detrusor contraction or an over-distended bladder (1). Although conservative methods of treatment are described for the treatment of GUSI, one of the most commonly used modalities is surgery (2). Since the introduction of the retropubic urethral suspension in 1910, over 100 different surgical techniques for the treatment of GUSI have been described (3).

The first retropubic technique for GUSI was described by Marshall, Marchetti and Krantz in 1949 (4). The technique fixed periurethral pubocervical fascia to the posterior pubic bone using sutures. They reported a success rate of 82%. In 1961, Burch described a modification of this technique by attaching the periurethral tissue to the iliopectineal line (Cooper's ligament) (5). He reported a success rate of 93% (6).

Emphasizing the principles of minimally invasive surgery, the laparoscopic approach has been successfully adopted for many procedures that previously relied on an open abdominal or transvaginal route. First described in 1991, the laparoscopic retropubic colposuspension gained popularity because of its reported advantages of improved visualization, shorter hospital stay, faster recovery and decreased blood loss (7). However, recent advances in minimally invasive slings including the tension-free transvaginal tape (TVT) and the tension-free transobturator tape (TOT) slings may be slowing or causing the laparoscopic Burch to lose its popularity.

OPERATIVE INDICATIONS

Laparoscopy should be considered only as a mode of abdominal access and not a change in the operative technique. Ideally, the indications for a laparoscopic approach to retropubic colposuspension should be the same as an open (laparotomy) approach. This would include patients with GUSI and urethral hypermobility. The authors believe that the laparoscopic Burch colposuspension can be substituted for an open Burch colposuspension in the majority of cases. Factors that might influence this decision include any history of previous pelvic or anti-incontinence surgery, the patient's age and weight, the need for concomitant surgery, contraindications to general anesthesia and the surgeon's experience. The surgeon's decision to proceed with a laparoscopic approach should be based on an objective clinical assessment of the patient as well as the surgeon's own surgical skills. If the patient demonstrates a cystocele secondary to a paravaginal defect diagnosed either pre-or intraoperatively, a paravaginal defect repair should be performed before the colposuspension. This approach combines the paravaginal repair with Burch colposuspension for treatment of anterior vaginal prolapse secondary to paravaginal defects and stress urine incontinence secondary to urethral hyper-mobility (3).

PREOPERATIVE CONSIDERATIONS

We recommend that all patients have a modified bowel preparation consisting of a full liquid diet 48 hours before scheduled surgery and a clear liquid diet and one bottle of magnesium citrate 24 hours before surgery. This regimen appears to improve visualization of the operative field by bowel decompression and reduces that chance of contamination in case of accidental bowel injury. A single dose of prophylactic intravenous antibiotics is administered 30 minutes before surgery. Anti-embolic compression stockings are routinely used. The patient is intubated, given general anesthesia and placed in a dorsal lithotomy position with both arms tucked to her side. A 16F three-way Foley catheter with a 5 ml balloon tip is inserted into the bladder and attached to continuous drainage.

SURGICAL TECHNIQUE

Laparoscopic Paravaginal Repair

We routinely perform open laparoscopy at the inferior margin of the umbilicus. A 10-mm access port is used at this site to introduce the laparoscope. The abdomen is insufflated with CO_2 to 15 mmHg intra-abdominal pressure. Three additional ports are placed under direct vision (Fig. 1.) The choice of the individual port size depends on what concomitant surgery is planned for that patient.

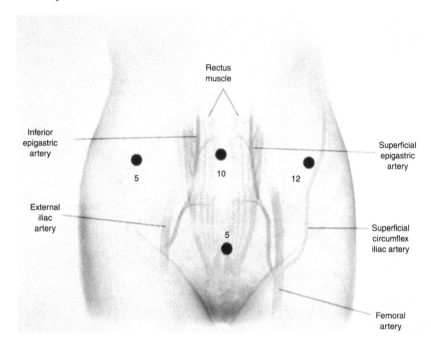

Figure 1 Port placement for laparoscopic Burch procedure.

The bladder is filled in a retrograde fashion with 200 to 300 mL normal saline, allowing identification of the superior border of the bladder edge. Entrance into the space of Retzius is accomplished by a transperitoneal approach using a harmonic scalpel. The incision is made approximately 3 cm above the bladder rejection, beginning along the medial border of the right obliterated umbilical ligament. Immediate identification of loose areolar tissue at the point of incision confirms a proper plane of dissection.

After the space of Retzius has been entered and the pubic ramus visualized, the bladder is drained to prevent injury. The retropubic space is developed by separating the loose areolar and fatty layers using blunt dissection. Blunt dissection is continued until the retropubic anatomy is visualized. The pubic symphysis and bladder neck are identified in the midline and the obturator neurovascular bundle, Cooper's ligament and the arcus tendineus fascia pelvis are visualized bilaterally along the pelvic sidewall (Fig. 2). The anterior vaginal wall and its point of lateral attachment from its origin at the pubic symphysis to its insertion at the ischial spine is identified. If paravaginal wall defects are present, the lateral margins of the pubocervical fascia will be detached from the pelvic sidewall at the arcus tendineus fascia pelvis (white line). The lateral margins of the detached pubocervical fascia and the broken edge of the white line can usually be

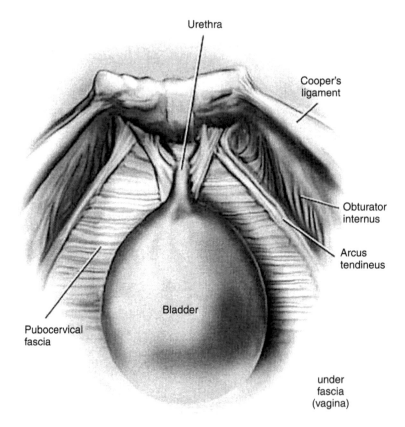

Urethra

Cooper's
ligament

Obturator
internus

Arcus
tendineus

Bladder

Pubocervical
fascia

under
fascia
(vagina)

Figure 2   Normal antomy: space of Retzius. *Source*: Courtesy of John R. Miklos.

clearly visualized confirming the paravaginal defect. Unilateral or bilateral
defects may be present (Fig. 3).

   We recommend completion of the laparoscopic paravaginal repair
before the colposuspension. After identification of the defect, the combined
repair is begun by inserting the surgeon's non-dominant hand into the
vagina to elevate the anterior vaginal wall and the pubocervical fascia to
their normal attachment along the arcus tendineus fascia pelvis. A 2-0 non-
absorbable suture with attached needle is introduced through the 12-mm
port, and the needle is grasped using a laparoscopic needle driver.

   The first suture is placed near the apex of the vagina through the
paravesical portion of the pubocervical fascia. The needle is then passed
through the ipsilateral obturator internus muscle and fascia around
the arcus tendineus fascia at its origin 1 to 2 cm distal to the ischial spine.
The suture is secured using an extracorporeal knot-tying technique. Good
tissue approximation is accomplished without a suture bridge. Sutures are

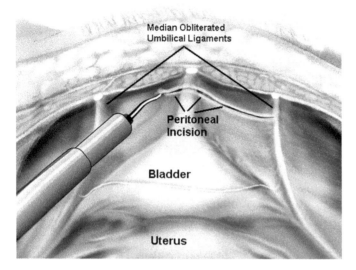

Figure 3 Entering the space of Retzius—a transperitoneal approach. *Source*: Courtesy of John R. Miklos.

placed sequentially along the paravaginal defects from the ischial spine towards the urethrovesical junction. Usually, a series of two to four sutures is placed between the ischial spine and a point 1 to 2 cm proximal to the urethrovesical junction (Fig. 4). The laparoscopic colposuspension is performed distal to the urethrovesical junction. The surgical procedure is repeated on the patient's opposite side if bilateral defects are present. Upon completion of the bilateral paravaginal repair, the Burch colposuspension is performed. By performing the paravaginal defect repair first, normal anatomic support of the anterior vaginal segment is recreated, reducing the chance of over-elevation of the paraurethral Burch sutures and subsequent voiding dysfunction.

Laparoscopic Burch Colposuspension

This laparoscopic technique parallels our open technique and has previously been described (8). The laparoscopic colposuspension is performed using non-absorbable (No. 0) sutures; we routinely use polytrifluoroethylene. The surgeon's non-dominant hand is placed in the vagina and a finger is used to elevate the vagina. The endopelvic fascia on both sides of the bladder neck and midurethra is exposed using an endoscopic blunt dissector. The first suture is placed 2 cm lateral to the urethra at the level of the midurethra. A figure of 8-suture, incorporating the entire thickness of the anterior vaginal wall excluding the epithelium, is taken, and the suture is then passed through the ipsilateral Cooper's ligament.

With an assistant's fingers in the vagina to elevate the anterior vaginal wall towards Cooper's ligament, the suture is tied down with a series of

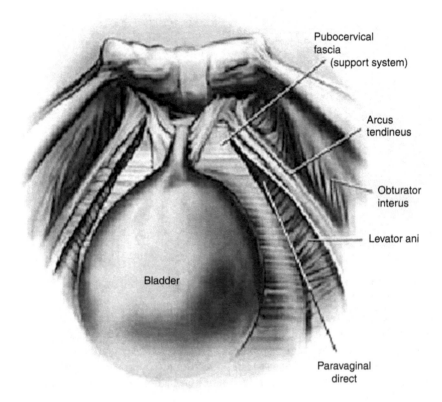

Figure 4 Paravaginal defects. Loss of lateral vaginal attachment at the arcus tendineus.

extracorporeal knots using an endoscopic knot pusher. An additional suture is then placed in a similar fashion at the level of the urethrovesical junction, approximately 2 cm lateral to the bladder edge on the same side. The procedure is repeated on the opposite side. Excessive tension on the vaginal wall should be avoided when tying down the sutures. We routinely leave a suture bridge of approximately of 2 to 3 cm (Fig. 5).

Upon completion of the paravaginal repair and Burch urethropexy, the intra-abdominal pressure is reduced to 10 to 12 mmHg, and the retropubic space is inspected for hemostasis. Cystoscopy is performed to rule out urinary tract injury. The patient is given 5 mL of indigo carmine and 10 mL furosemide intravenously, and a 70-degree cystoscope is used to visualize the bladder lumen, assess for un-intentional stitch penetration and confirm bilateral ureteral patency. After cystoscopy, attention is returned to laparoscopy. We recommend routine closure of the anterior peritoneal defect using a multifire hernia stapler. All ancillary trocar sheaths are removed under direct vision to ensure hemostasis and exclude iatrogenic bowel herniation. Excess gas is

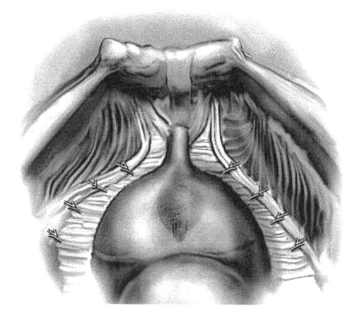

Figure 5   Paravaginal defect repair. Reattachment of vagina laterally to the arcus tendineus.

expelled and fascial defects of 10 mm or more are closed using delayed absorbable suture. Postoperative bladder drainage and voiding trials are accomplished either using a transurethral catheter, suprapubic tube or intermittent self-catheterization.

CLINICAL RESULTS

Since Vancaillie and Schuessler published the first laparoscopic colposuspension case series in 1991, many other investigators have reported their experience. Review of the literature reveals a lack of uniformity in surgical technique and surgical materials used for colposuspension. This lack of standardization is also noted with the conventional open (laparotomy) technique. Because of this lack of standardization and the steep learning curve associated with laparoscopic suturing, surgeons have attempted to develop faster and easier ways of performing a laparoscopic Burch colposuspension. These modifications have included the use of stapling devices (9), bone anchors (10), synthetic mesh (11–13) and fibrin glue (13,14). However, we believe that the laparoscopic approach should be identical with the open technique to allow comparative studies.

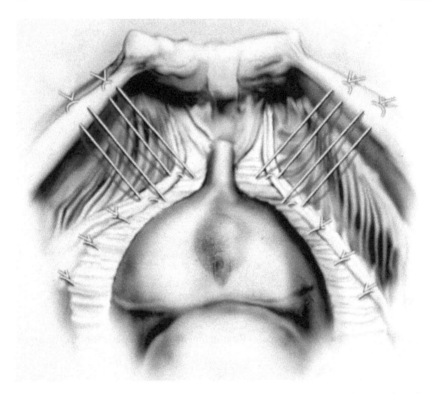

Figure 6 Paravaginal repair and Burch procedure. A combined operation for correction of the cystocele and urinary stress incontinence.

There are many reported laparoscopic Burch colposuspension case series that have used conventional surgical technique and suture materials. Published cure rates range from 58 to 100%, with the majority of the studies reporting cure rates greater than 80% (Table 1) (15–54).

Although there have been no studies regarding the long-term results of the laparoscopic paravaginal plus Burch colposuspension procedure, one would assume that there is a higher cure rate for the paravaginal plus Burch colposuspension (8 to 12 sutures) compared with the Burch colposuspension only (four sutures) for the treatment of urinary stress incontinence, because more sutures results in a greater distribution of force to the pelvic floor during episodes of increased abdominal pressure (Fig. 6).

Most authors have reported decreased blood loss, shortened hospitalization and decreased postoperative pain and recovery time. Our experience of 171 laparoscopic paravaginal repair and Burch urethropexy procedures has seen an average operative time of 70 min, hospital stays of less than 23 h, estimated blood loss of less than 50 mL and an overall lower urinary tract

Table 1 Published Cure Rates of Laparoscopic Burch Procedures

Author (year)	No. of patients	Follow-up (mo)	Objective data	Cure rate (%)
Albala et al. (1992)	10	7	Yes	100[a]
Burton (1993)	30	12		73
Liu (1993)	58	22	Yes	94.8
Liu and Paek (1993)	107	18	Yes	97.2
Polascik et al. (1994)	12	20.8		83
Liu (1994)	132	18	Yes	96
Gunn et al. (1994)	15	4–9	Yes	100
Nezhat et al. (1994)	62	8–30	Yes	100[a]
Carter (1995)	30	18		100
Lam et al. (1995)	15	9		100
Lyons (1995)	10	>12		90[a]
McDougal et al. (1995)	10	12		78[a]
Ross (1995)	32	12	Yes	94
Langebrekke et al. (1995)	8	3	Yes	94
Radomski et al. (1995)	34	17.3		85
Das and Palmer (1995)	10	10		90[a]
Flax (1996)	47	8.2		73[a]
Karabacak et al. (1996)	35	12		100[a]
Ross (1996)	35	12	Yes	91
Cooper et al. (1996)	113	8		87
Lam et al. (1997)	107	16	Yes	91
Su et al. (1997)	46	12	Yes	80[a]
Burton (1997)	30	36	Yes	60
Papasakelariou and Papasakelariou (1997)	32	24		91
Lobel and Davis (1997)	35	34		69[a]
Lee et al. (1998)	48	26	Yes	93.8
Ross (1998)	48	24	Yes	89
Miannay et al. (1998)	36	24		69
Saidi et al. (1998)	70	15.9		91[a]
Persson and Wolner-Hanssen (2000)	78	12	Yes	58[a]
Persson and Wolner-Hanssen (2000)	83	12	Yes	83
Lee et al. (2001)	150	>36		90.7
Moore et al. (2001)	33	18.6	Yes	90
Ross et al. (2001)	46	12	Yes	93
Zullo et al. (2001)	30	12	Yes	89
Cosson et al. (2002)	74	12		97
Chung and Chung (2002)	51	12	Yes	100

(Continued)

Table 1   Published Cure Rates of Laparoscopic Burch Procedures (*Continued*)

Author (year)	No. of patients	Follow-up (mo)	Objective data	Cure rate (%)
Ustun et al. (2003)	23	13.5	Yes	82.6
Paraiso et al. (2004)	33	12	Yes	81
Dietz and Wilson (2004)	50	12		74
Huang and Yang (2004)	82	12		89

[a] Some or all Burch procedures were performed with one suture on each side of the urethra.

injury rate of less than 3% without an incidence of urethral compromise. Although some have reported subsequent laparotomy to repair the cystotomy, in all cases we have been able to repair the bladder laparoscopically. This is performed using a delayed absorbable suture in an interrupted single-layer fashion. Because all cystotomies were found in the dome of the bladder, prolonged bladder catheterization was not necessary. The Foley catheter was removed when the patient could empty 80% of her total bladder volume. Early recognition of bladder injury and proficiency in laparoscopic suturing techniques are critical elements in this approach. Reports suggest this complication depends on the learning curve and declines with increasing surgical experience (55).

CONCLUSION

Despite its recent introduction and lack of long-term data, the laparoscopic Burch colposuspension has become popular for treatment of urinary stress incontinence. Although initial data suggest that this technique is a safe and effective alternative to traditional laparotomy, surgeons should approach it with caution. Laparoscopic suturing and a thorough knowledge of anatomy are essential if we are to have long-term outcome data equivalent to the traditional open technique. Future prospective randomized clinical trials may establish the laparoscopic approach as a minimally invasive method for successful long-term treatment of genuine anatomic urinary stress incontinence as well as anterior vaginal segment prolapse.

REFERENCES

1. Fantl J, Newman D, Coling J, et al. Urinary incontinence in adults: Acute and chronic management. Clinical Practice Guidelines, No. 2, 1996 Update. Rockville, MD: U.S. Department of Health and Human Services. Public Health Service, Agency for Health Care Policy and Research. AHCPR Publication No. 96-0682. March 1996: 1996.

2. Buller JL, Cundiff GW. Laparoscopic surgeries for urinary incontinence. Clin Obstet Gynecol 2000; 43(3):604–18.
3. Miklos JR, Kohli N. "Paravaginal Plus" Burch procedure: a laparoscopic approach. J Pelvic Surg 1998; 4:297–302.
4. Marshall V, Marchetti A, Krantz K. The correction of stress incontinence by simple vesicourethral suspension. Surg Gynecol Obstet 1949; 88:509–18.
5. Burch J. Urethrovaginal fixation to Cooper's ligament for correction of stress incontinence, cystocele and prolapse. Am J Obstet Gyencol 1961; 81:281–90.
6. Burch J. Cooper's ligament urethrovesicle suspension for stress incontinence. Am J Obstet Gyencol 1968; 100:764–74.
7. Vancaille TG, Schussler W. Laparoscopic bladder-neck suspension. J Laparoendosc Surg 1991; 1:169–73.
8. Kohli N, Miklos JR. Laparoscopic Burch colposuspension: a modern approach. Contem Obstet Gynecol 1997; 42:36–55.
9. Ou CS, Presthus J, Beadle E. Laparoscopic bladder neck suspension using hernia mesh and surgical staples. J Laparoendosc Surg 1993; 3:563–6.
10. Takeda M, Hatano A, Kurumada S, et al. Bladder neck suspension using percutaneous bladder neck stabilization to the pubic bone with a bone-anchor suture fixation system: a new extraperitoneal laparoscopic approach. Urol Int 1999; 62:57–60.
11. Von Theobald P, Levy G. Laparoscopic preperitoneal colposuspension for stress incontinence in women. Surg Endosc 1995; 9:1189–92.
12. Hannah S. Chin A. Laparoscopic retropubic urethropexy. J Am Assoc Gynecol Laparosc 1996; 4:47–52.
13. Manhes H. Laparoscopic Retzio-plasty. A new surgical approach to stress incontinence. Int Surg 1996; 81:371–3.
14. Kiilholma P, Haarala M, Polvi H, Makinen J, Chancellor M. Sutureless endoscopic colposuspension with fibrin sealant. Tech Urol 1995; 1:81–3.
15. Albala DM, Schuessler WW, Vancaillie TG. Laparoscopic bladder suspension for the treatment of stress incontinence. Semin Urol 1992; 10:222–5.
16. Burton G. A randomized comparison of laparoscopic and open colposuspension (abstract). Neurourol Urodyn 1993; 16:353–4.
17. Liu C. Laparoscpic retropubic colposuspension (Burch procedure): a review of 58 cases. J Reprod Med 1993; 38:526–30.
18. Liu C, Paek W. Laparoscopic retropubic colposuspension (Burch procedure). J Am Assoc Gyencol Laparosc 1993; 1:31–5.
19. Polascik TJ, Moore RG, Rosenberg MT, Kavoussi LR. Comparison of laparoscopic and open retropubic colposuspension for treatment of urinary stress incontinence. Urology 1995; 45:647–52.
20. Liu CY. Laparoscopic treatment of genuine urinary stress incontinence. Clin Obstet Gynecol 1994; 8:789–98.
21. Gunn GC, Cooper RP, Gordon NS, Gragnon L. Use of a new device for endoscopic suturing in the laparoscopic Burch procedure. J Am Assoc Gynecol Laparoscopists 1994; 2:65–70.
22. Nezhat CH, Nezhat F, Nezhat CR et al. Laparoscopic retropubic cystocolposuspension. J Am Assoc Gynecol Laparoscopists 1994; 1:339–49.
23. Carter J. Laparoscopic bladder neck suspension. Endo Surg 1995; 3:81–7.

24. Lam A, Jenkins G, Hyslop R. Laparoscopic Burch colposuspension for stress incontinence: preliminary results. Med J Aust 1995; 162:18–21.

25. Lyons TL, Winer WK. Clinical outcomes with laparoscopic approaches and open Burch procedures for urinary stress incontinence. J Am Assoc Gynecol Laparoscopists 1995; 2:193–7.

26. McDougal EM, Klutke CG, Cornell T. Comparison of transvaginal versus laparoscopic bladder neck suspension for urinary stress incontinence. Adult Urol 1995; 45:641–5.

27. Ross JW. Laparoscopic Burch repair compared to laparotomy Burch for cure of urinary stress incontinence. Int Urogyneecol 1995; 6:323–8.

28. Langebrekke A, Dahlstrom B, Eraker R, Urnes A. The laparoscopic Burch procedure: a preliminary report. Acta Obstet Gynecol Scand 1995; 74:153–5.

29. Radomski SB, Herschorn S. Laparoscopic Burch bladder neck suspension: early results. J Urol 1996; 155:515–8.

30. Das S, Palmer J. Laparoscopic colposuspenison. J Urol 1995; 154:1119–21.

31. Flax S. The gasless laparoscopic Burch bladder neck suspension: early experience. J Urol 1996; 156:1105–7.

32. Karabacak O, Taner M, Tiras M, Kaya A, Guner H, Yildirim M. An extraperitoneal Burch procedure: a case report. J Laparoendosc Surg 1996; 6: 65–8.

33. Ross JW. Two techniques of laparoscopic Burch repair for stress incontinence: a prospective randomized study. J Am Assoc Gynecol Laparoscopists 1996; 3:351–7.

34. Cooper MJ, Cario G, Lam A, Carolton M. A review of results in a series of 113 laparoscopic colposuspensions. Aust NZJ Obstet Gynaecol 1996; 36:44–9.

35. Lam AM, Jenkins GJ, Hyslop RS. Laparoscopic Burch colposuspension for stress incontinence: preliminary results. Med J Aust 1995; 162:18–22.

36. Su TH, Wang KG, Hsu CY, Wei H, Hong BK. Prospective comparison of laparoscopic and traditional colposuspensions in the treatment of genuine stress incontinence. Acta Obstet Gynecol 1997; 76:576–82.

37. Burton G. A three-year prospective randomized urodynamic study comparing open and laparoscopic colposuspension (Abstract). Neurourol Urodyn 1997; 16:353–4.

38. Papasakelariou C, Papasakelariou B. Laparoscopic bladder neck suspension. J Am Assoc Gynecol Laparoscopists 1997; 4:185–8.

39. Lobel RW, Davis GD. Long-term results of laparoscopic Burch colposuspension. J Am Assoc Gyencol Laparoscopists 1997; 4:341–5.

40. Lee C, Yen C, Want C, Huang K, Soong Y. Extraperitoneoscopic colposuspension using CO_2 distension method. Int Surg 1998; 83:262–4.

41. Ross J. Multichannel urodynamic evaluation of laparoscopic Burch colposuspension for genuine stress incontinence. Obstet Gynecol 1998; 91:55–9.

42. Miannay E, Cosson M, Querleu D, Crepin G. Comparison etre la colposuspension par coelioscopie et laprotomi dans le traitement de l'incontinence urinaire d'effort. Etude comparative a partir de 72 cas apparies. Contracept Fertil Sex 1998; 26:376–85.

43. Saidi MH, Gallagher MS, Skop IP et al. Extraperitoneal laparoscopic colposuspension: short-term cure rate, complications and duration of hospital stay comparison with Burch colposuspension. Obstet Gynecol 1998; 92:619–25.

44. Persson J, Wolner-Hanssen P. Laparoscopic Burch colposuspension for urinary stress incontinence; a randomized comparison of one or two sutures on each side of the urethra. Obstet Gynecol 2000; 95:151–5.
45. Lee Cl, Yen CF, Wang CJ, Hain S, Soong YK. Extraperitoneal approach to laparoscopic Burch colposuspension. J Am Assoc Gynecol Laparosc 2001; 8(3): 374–7.
46. Moore RD, Speights SE, Miklos JR. Laparoscopic Burch colposuspension for recurrent urinary stress incontinence. J Am Assoc Gynecol Laparosc 2001; 8(3): 389–92.
47. Ross JW. Laparoscopic Burch colposuspension and overlapping schincteroplasty for double incontinence. JSLS 2001; 5(3):203–9.
48. Zullo F, Plaomba S, Piccione F, Morelli M, Arduino B, Mastrantonio P. Laparoscopic Burch colposuspension: a randomized controlled trial comparing two transperitoneal surgical techniques. Obstet Gynecol 2001; 98(5 Pt 1):783–8.
49. Cosson M, Rajabally R, Bogaert E, Querleu D, Crepin G. Laparoscopic sacrocolpopexy, hysterectomy, and burch colposuspension: feasibility and short-term complications of 77 procedures. JSLS 2002; 6(2):1115–9.
50. Chung MK, Chung R. Comparison of Laparoscopic Burch and Tension-Free vaginal tape in treating urinary stress incontinence in obese patients. JSLS 2002; 6:17–21.
51. Ustun Y, Engin-Ustun Y, Gungor M, Tezcan S. Tension-free vaginal tape compared with laparoscopic Burch urethropexy. J Am Assoc Gynecol Laparosc 2003; 10(3):386–9.
52. Paraiso MF, Wlaters MD, Karram MM, Barber MD. Laparoscopic burch colposuspension versus tension-free vaginal tape: a randomized trial. Obstet Gynecol 2004; 104(6):1249–58.
53. Dietz HP, Wilson PD. Laparoscopic colposuspension versus urthropexy: a case–control series. Int Urogyncol J Pelvic Floor Dysfunct 2005; 16(1): 15–18Au: Please provide publication details for Ref. (53) if any.
54. Huang WC, Yang JM. Anatomic comparison between laparoscopic and open Burch colposuspension for primary urinary stress incontinence. Urology 2004; 63(4):678–81.
55. Miklos JR and Kohli N. Laparoscopic paravaginal repair plus Burch colposuspension: review and descriptive technique. Urology 2000; 56. Supple 6A:64–6.

6

Surgical Techniques for Synthetic Suburethral Sling Placement: TVT and TOT

Renaud de Tayrac

Groupe Hospitalier Caremeau, Service de Gynécologie-Obstétrique du Pr Mares, Nîmes, France

Hervé Fernandez

Service de Gynécologie-Obstétrique et d'Histologie-Embryologie-Cytogénétique à orientation Biologique et Génétique de la Reproduction, Hôpital Antoine Béclère, Assistance Publique-Hôpitaux de Paris, Clamart, France

INTRODUCTION

Urinary stress incontinence (USI) is a common functional disorder occurring in women. A large number of surgical procedures have been designed for the treatment of female USI. The rationale of the surgical treatment of USI has totally changed over the past 10 years, because the techniques using urethral suspension were responsible for acute urinary retention and chronic voiding troubles. New techniques to support the urethra and the anterior vaginal wall have been developed.

The tension-free vaginal tape procedure (TVT) has been used in the treatment of female USI since 1995 (1). Although TVT has a high long-term success rate, ranging from 85% to 95% (2–4), there have been concerns regarding its operative safety in relation to bowel and major blood vessel injuries, bladder and urethral perforation, and post-operative urgency and voiding difficulties.

In 2001, the transobturator surgical approach (TOT) was introduced for the placement of suburethral tapes, with the aim of sparing the retropubic space (5). Clinical results as well as anatomical work have suggested that this approach may be safer. In 2003, a modified transobturator approach was described, in which the tape is inserted from the suburethral incision to the skin incisions (TVT-O).

TENSION-FREE VAGINAL TAPE

Background

Tension-free vaginal tape (TVT) was introduced in 1995 as a minimally invasive technique for surgical correction of female urinary stress incontinence, under local anesthesia and on ambulatory basis. First described in Sweden by Ulmsten and Petros (1), the TVT has been used extensively all over the world following clinical trials that established its safety and effectiveness.

The procedure is based on the concept of the suburethral sling, but many studies have suggested that the TVT is associated with a higher success rate than previous sling procedures and a significantly lower incidence of intraoperative and post-operative complications. The procedure is usually performed by vaginal route under local or regional anesthesia, on ambulatory basis with a hospital stay of less than 24 hours. In addition, the learning curve of the procedure is short and outcomes seem to be uniform and independent of operator bias. These characteristics make the procedure ideally suited for patients with USI due to urethral hyper mobility and/or intrinsic sphincter deficiency.

Instrumentation

The TVT instrumentation consists of a reusable stainless steel introducer, a reusable rigid catheter guide, and the TVT device, which is a single-use apparatus composed of a 1×40 cm strip of polypropylene mesh (Prolene, Ethicon) covered by a plastic sheath and held between two stainless steel needles (Fig. 1). The plastic sheath is designed to cover the synthetic mesh during placement of the sling and thereby reduce the incidence of contamination, post-operative infection that may result in graft rejection, and to allow easy passage of the tape. The tape is configured to stay fixed in place once the smooth protective cover is removed, before completion of the procedure.

Surgical Technique

The procedure includes the following steps:

1. The patient is placed in the dorsal lithotomy position with her hips flexed no more than 90° over the abdomen and her buttocks positioned flush with the edge of the operating table.
2. The TVT procedure can be performed under various forms of anesthesia, depending on patient preference and the need for concurrent surgical procedures. It is recommended that the procedure

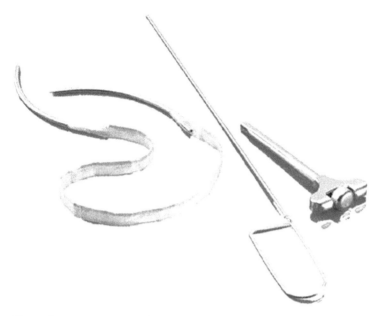

Figure 1   Tension-free vaginal tape instrumentation: introducer, catheter guide, and polypropylene mesh covered by a plastic sheath.

initially be performed under local anesthesia with intravenous sedation so that a cough stress test could be performed intraoperatively. The stress test permits proper adjustment of the tape, and thus maximizes efficacy and minimizes post-operative voiding dysfunction.

3. The operative field is prepared with a standard antiseptic agent and the patient draped taking care to keep the suprapubic region in the operative field and the anus covered.

4. The bladder is emptied with a Foley catheter. The rigid guide is inserted into the Foley catheter to facilitate identification of the urethra and the bladder neck during passage of the introducers.

5. The desired exit points of the introducers are marked with two 5 mm skin incisions, placed 1 cm above the pubic symphysis and at 2 cm lateral to the midline, on each side.

6. A posterior vaginal retractor is inserted into the vagina, to expose the anterior vaginal wall. Using gentle traction on the Foley catheter to identify the location of the bladder neck, 10 ml of local anesthetic or saline (for patients under regional or general anesthesia) is injected into the vaginal mucosa and submucosal tissues in the midline and bilaterally at the level of the mid urethra, in order to prepare the dissection space.

7. A 10 to 15 mm sagittal incision is made in the midline of the anterior vaginal wall approximately 10 mm below the external urethral meatus.

The edges of this incision are grasped using Allis clamps, and minimal dissection is used to free the vaginal wall from the urethra and develop a small paraurethral space bilaterally, using curved scissors. The path of the lateral dissection should be orientated at a 30° angle from the midline sagittal plane, with the tips pointed slightly upward. The dissection is continued toward the inferior edge of the body of the pubic bone, between the pubic symphysis and the inferior pubic ramus. It is not necessary to perforate the endopelvic fascia with the scissors. The introducers are inserted through the vaginal incision.

8. To minimize the risk of bladder or urethral perforation during this process, the handle of the guide within the Foley catheter is first moved to the ipsilateral side.

9. Before placement of the tape, the introducer is attached to one of the stainless steel needles and the retractor is removed from the vagina. The shaft of the introducer is grasped and the tip of the needle is inserted into the previously developed paraurethral space until it reaches the endopelvic fascia. Then, the endopelvic fascia is perforated just behind the inferior surface of the pubic bone. On entry into the retropubic space, the needle is guided up to the abdominal incision, maintaining contact with the back of the pubic bone (Fig. 2); this

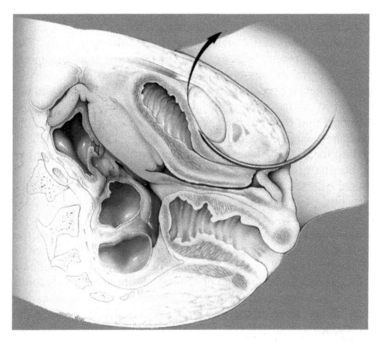

Figure 2 TVT technique. Into the retropubic space, the needle is guided up to the abdominal incision, maintaining contact with the back of the pubic bone.

minimizes the risk of vascular or hollow viscous injury. A second layer of resistance is felt as the needle passes through the muscular and fascial layers of the abdominal wall. Passage of the needle is completed once the tip passes through the small abdominal incision on the ipsilateral side.

10. Before complete extraction of the needle through the suprapubic incision, unintentional bladder perforation must be excluded. The rigid catheter guide is removed and the bladder emptied through the indwelling catheter. The catheter is removed and a 70° cystoscope is used to confirm bladder integrity. If a bladder perforation is noted, generally on the upper lateral side of the bladder wall, the needle is removed by pulling the introducer, following which the insertion procedure is repeated, making certain that the needle stays *in contact with the back of the pubic bone* and ensuring its direction is not too lateral. Once correct placement has been confirmed by repeat cystoscopy, the needle is detached from the introducer and pulled through the abdominal incision.

11. This technique is repeated in an identical fashion on the contra lateral side, making certain the tape lies flat against the suburethral tissue at the level of the mid urethra. Then the plastic sheath covering the tape is completely pulled through the skin until the tape appears.

12. The tape is positioned loosely e.g., without tension, and flat under the urethra. The cough stress test is performed at this stage. This allows adjustment of the tape so that only a few drops of urine are lost during the coughing process. When the tape is in its final position (Fig. 3), the plastic sheathing that covers the tapes is removed. During this step, a blunt instrument (e.g., scissors or forceps) is placed between the urethra and the tape to prevent an increase in the tension of the tape.

13. The vaginal incision is closed; the ends of the tape are cut bilaterally at their exit points just below the skin. The skin incisions are closed with a suture or surgical adhesive tape. Routine use of prophylactic intravenous antibiotics is recommended.

14. The indwelling urinary catheter is left in place and removed within the first 24 hours. After removal of the catheter post-void residuals are checked by intermittent catheterization or via ultrasonographic assessment of the bladder.

The majority of these patients experience minimal discomfort; adequate pain control is achieved with use of non-opioid oral medication. Most are discharged within the first 24 hours after surgery. Before discharge, the patient is given detailed instructions and post-operative recommendations together with a handout containing the same information. Patients usually resume their normal daily activities within 1 to 2 weeks after the procedure but are cautioned to avoid heavy lifting and strenuous exercise for up to 6

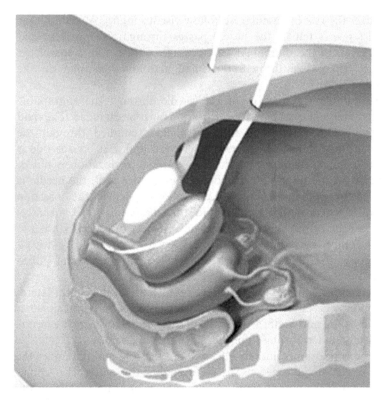

Figure 3 TVT technique: Position of the tape should be loose and flat under the urethra.

weeks postoperatively to allow adequate healing. Patients also are instructed to abstain from sexual intercourse and avoid tampon use during the same period and return for a follow-up visit in 6 weeks.

Clinical Data

More than 500,000 such procedures performed in the world have confirmed the long term results reported by Ulmsten (1): success in 85%, improvement in 10%, and failure in 5% (2–4). Use of the TVT has been demonstrated to also be effective for mixed urinary incontinence (6) and in recurrent urinary stress incontinence (7). Nevertheless, the efficacy in patients with intrinsic sphincter deficiency is inferior with a success rate of 75%, improvement in 10%, and failure in 15% (8).

A prospective randomized study between open Burch colposuspension and TVT has shown similar continence rates at 2 years follow-up (9). Another study has shown similar continence rates between laparoscopic Burch colposuspension and TVT (10); TVT was associated with the advantages of reduced operative time and length of post-operative recovery period. In addition, there no cases of posterior compartment prolapse after TVT, as opposed to with colposuspension (11).

Despite the simplicity, reproducibility and high long-term success rates associated with the TVT procedure, there are concerns regarding its operative safety. Most of the series have reported a 5% to 10% risk of bladder perforation associated with the placement of the stainless steel introducers. The other common complication has been hematoma of the retropubic space. The reported major operative complications include: bowel injuries (12) and major blood vessels injuries resulting in death (13).

To avoid the major injuries mentioned, one of the approaches suggested is the insertion of the introducers from the suprapubic skin incisions to the suburethral space by an abdominal retropubic approach. A randomized comparison with the TVT has shown similar continence rates, but a higher rate of urethral injury with the abdominal approach (4.9% *vs.* 0%) (14).

Post-operative voiding troubles, such as voiding difficulties and urgency, occur in 5% to 15% of TVT patients (2–4,15,16). The rate of voiding difficulties is correlated to the tension applied to the tape. Although preoperative urgency is improved in 60% to 70% of the patients after TVT, there are no preoperative parameters that can predict the outcome.

Complications specifically associated with the use of synthetic materials, such as graft rejection, fistula formation, abscess or hypersensitivity reactions have been exceptionally reported with the use of monofilament polypropylene tapes such as the TVTs. However, we must remind the reader that graft rejection and vaginal erosion occurs in up to 9% of cases in which multifilament tapes are used (17).

Conclusion

The TVT is a relatively safe and effective, minimally invasive surgical technique for the treatment of female urinary stress incontinence. It is associated with a short learning curve. Clinical studies have demonstrated the TVT cure rates to be comparable to more invasive procedures, such as open and laparoscopic Burch colposuspension. However, concerns remain regarding its safety; due to the intra-operative complications mentioned above.

TRANSOBTURATOR TAPE

Background

In 2001, the French urologist E. Delorme introduced the transobturator approach for the application of a tape (5). In Delorme's technique, the tunneler is introduced from the skin incisions, placed 2 cm lateral to the fold of the thigh, to the vaginal incision. The introducer passes through the obturator foramen (external obturator muscle, obturator membrane, internal obturator muscle) as is described further. The originality of that technique is the trajectory of the tape; it avoids the pelvic region, it reproduces the natural support of the urethra by the pubo-urethral ligaments (Fig. 4).

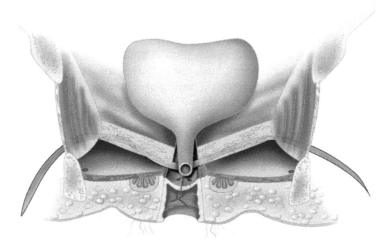

Figure 4   TOT placement: the perineal position of the mesh avoids the pelvic region and reproduces the natural support of the urethra by the pubo-urethral ligaments.

Instrumentation

The "tunneller" is a specially designed, curved needle (Fig. 5) similar to the Emmet needle. Its shape allows it to be turned around the ischio-pubic bone, from the skin incision to the suburethral incision, through the obturator foramen.

The tape is a monofilament of polypropylene, with a low elasticity (Obtape-LG®, Mentor-Porgès, le Plessis-Robinson, France). This tape is not covered by a plastic sheath.

Surgical Technique

The procedure includes the following steps:

1. The patient is placed in the dorsal lithotomy position with the hips hyperflexed over the abdomen (±110°). The buttocks are positioned flush with the edge of the operating table.
2. The procedure can be carried out under local, regional, or general anesthesia.

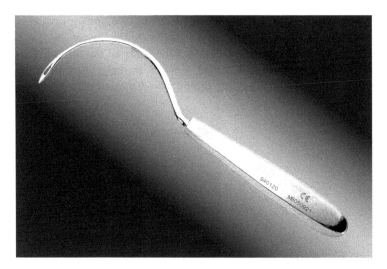

Figure 5   TOT instrumentation: the curved tuneller.

3. The operative field is prepared with a standard antiseptic agent and the patient draped, keeping the groin folds exposed and the anus covered.
4. An indwelling urethral catheter is inserted into the bladder, which is emptied.
5. A 15 mm sagittal midline incision is made through the vaginal mucosa starting 1cm below the urethral meatus (Fig. 6). This step may be

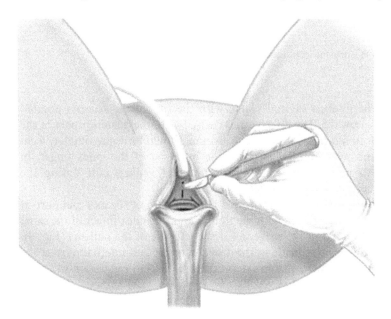

Figure 6   TOT surgical technique: suburethral incision.

preceded by sub-mucosal infiltration of 5 to 10 ml of saline (or lidocaine for procedures under local anesthesia) to facilitate the dissection.

6. The para-urethral subvaginal dissection is then carried out laterally, on both sides, using pointed and curved scissors, on both sides (Fig. 7). The path of the lateral dissection should be orientated at a 45° angle

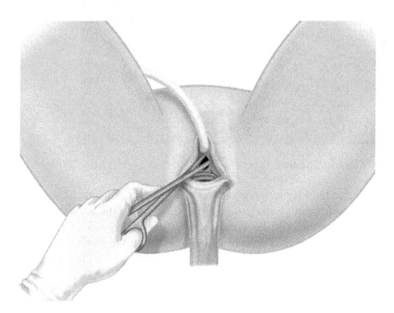

Figure 7   TOT surgical technique: para-urethral dissection.

from the midline sagittal plane, with the tips of the scissors pointed slightly upward. The dissection is carried until the posterior part of the inferior ischio-pubic ramus. The channel should be approximately 4 cm deep and wide enough to allow the insertion of the index finger, in order to protect the bladder, urethra and vaginal cuff during the introduction of the tunneller.

7. The obturator region is identified by palpation of the external part of the ischio-pubic ramus with the thumb and the index finger of the same hand (left hand of the surgeon for the left side of the patient) (Fig. 8).

8. A 5 mm incision is made in front of the upper and internal part of the obturator foramen, 15 mm lateral from the ischio-pubic ramus, at the level of the clitoris (Fig. 9).

9. The curved tunneller is inserted through the skin incision toward the obturator foramen. Perforation of the membrane is recognized from the

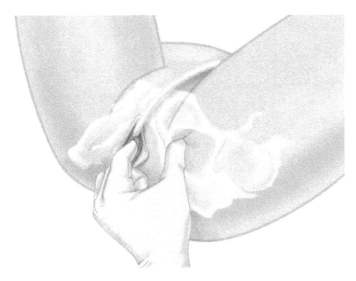

Figure 8   TOT surgical technique: palpation of the obturator region.

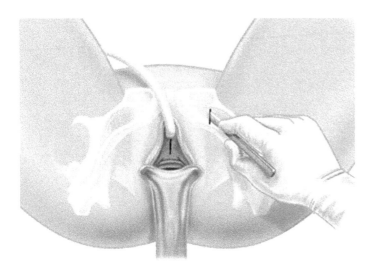

Figure 9   TOT surgical technique: skin incision, 15 mm outside of the ischio-pubic ramus.

resistance encountered in the process (Fig. 10). The index finger is placed into the ipsilateral para-urethral channel created earlier; the tunneller is turned around the ischio-pubic ramus, taking care to keep it in contact with the back side of the bone, until the tip of the tunneller reaches the finger (Fig. 11). The blind part of the procedure, e.g., the distance between

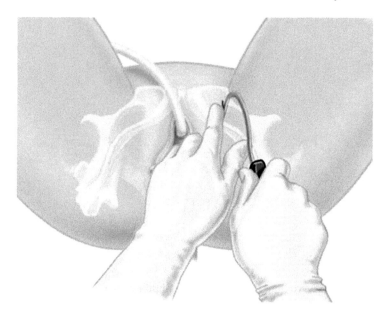

Figure 10   TOT surgical technique: perforation of the obturator membrane.

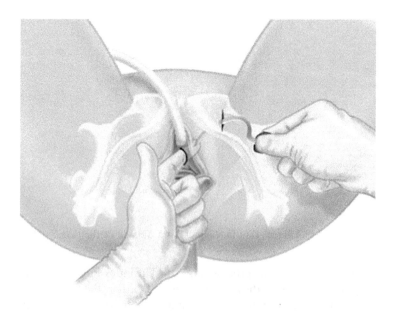

Figure 11   TOT surgical technique: movement of the tunneller around the ischio-pubic ramus and junction between the tip of the tunneller and the index finger.

the obturator membrane and the finger is normally less than 15 mm. Before the placement of the tape, the vagina must be inspected to ensure that it has not been perforated. If the blind part is more than 15 mm, or if there is an involuntary vaginal perforation, the tunneller must be pulled back to the level of the back side of the ischio-pubic ramus, and the procedure repeated.

10. When the tip of the tunneller is in contact with the finger, the tunneller is pushed through the channel to the suburethral space, keeping a permanent contact between device and the finger. Then, one end of the tape is attached onto the tip of the tunneller that came out of the vaginal incision, and pulled back through the previous trajectory of the tunneller and out of the skin incision (Fig. 12).

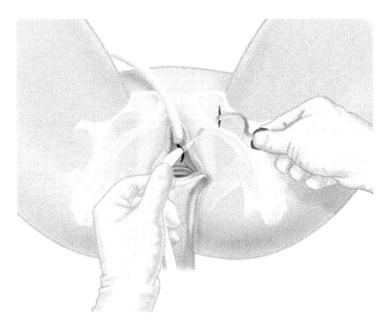

Figure 12 TOT surgical technique: the tape is connected with the tunneller and pulled outside through the obturator foramen.

During this process it may necessary to grasp the opposite vaginal edge with an Allis clamp, in order to stabilize the urethra.

11. The procedure is repeated on the collateral side making sure that the tape lies flat under the urethra. The tape is positioned loosely (without tension), and flat under the urethra. At this stage a cough test may be performed. This allows adjustment of the tape so that only a few drops

of urine are lost during the cough. To avoid the positioning the tape with excessive tension, a blunt instrument (e.g., scissors or forceps) is placed between the urethra and the tape during the adjustment (Fig. 13).

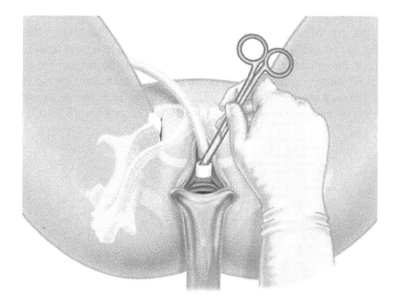

Figure 13   TOT surgical technique: adjustment of the tape should be loose and flat under the urethra, placing scissors between the urethra and the tape.

12. When the extremities of the tape have been extracted through both skin incisions, the protruding ends are cut just below the skin (Fig. 14).
13. Thereafter the vaginal incision is closed with interrupted absorbable sutures and the skin incisions are sutured or the edges apposed with surgical adhesive.
14. A cystoscopy is normally not indicated in the absence of operative difficulties. This is obviously dependent on the discretion of the surgeon.
15. A Foley catheter is left in place and removed within the first 24 post-operative hours. Thereafter, post-void residuals are measured by intermittent catheterization or bladder ultrasonography. Most patients experience minimal discomfort, and adequate pain control is achieved using oral nonopioid medications. Most patients are discharged within 24 hours after surgery. Before discharge, the patient is given detailed instructions and post-operative recommendations together with a handout containing the same information.

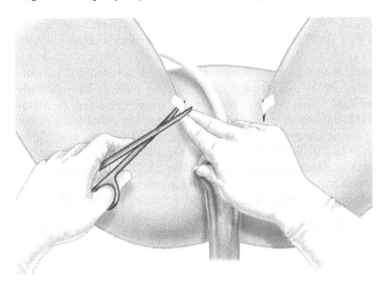

Figure 14   TOT surgical technique: the ends of the tape are cut just below the skin.

Patients usually resume their normal daily activities within 1 to 2 weeks, but are cautioned to avoid heavy lifting and strenuous exercise for up to 6 weeks post-operatively to allow adequate healing. Patients also are instructed to abstain from sexual intercourse and avoid tampon use for the same period and return for a follow-up visit in 6 weeks.

Clinical Data

More than 25,000 such procedures have been performed in the world. The preliminary results from Delorme (5) were confirmed by several series. At one year follow-up, the success rate is 80% to 90%, improvement 7% to 9% and failure 0% to 7% (18–20).

The mean operative time is about 15 minutes. The risk of intra-operative bladder injury is small (<0.5%). The rate of post-operative voiding dysfunction or de novo urge symptoms are 3.3% and 5%, respectively (20). There have been no reports of vascular, neurological or bowel injury. Nevertheless, infections were reported with the Uratape (Mentor-Porgès, Le Plessis-Robinson, France). One infected obturator hematoma (21) and one inguinal abscess have been reported (22); both infections occurred after vaginal erosion. The characteristics of the initial transobturator tape (woven and with a silicone patch under the urethra) were probably factors that contributed to these complications.

A retrospective nonrandomized study has been reported by Mellier et al., with the nonwoven tape. The cure rates were similar to those of the

TVT (90% and 95%, respectively). Bladder injuries were significantly greater with TVT (10% *vs.* 0%) as were hemorrhagic complications (10% *vs.* 2%) (23).

A French prospective multicenter registry had included 602 patients from November 2001 to September 2004 (24). All patients had clinically demonstrated USI with a positive pre-operative cough stress test. In 508 of these, the TOT was the sole procedure performed; the other 94 required concomitant repair for prolapse. The mean age of the patients was 57.3% years (range 29 to 88). The cohort of patients consisted of a heterogeneous and unselected population, since 21.2%, 35%, 11.5% and 26.9% of the patients enrolled had associated pre-operative urgency, mixed incontinence, low maximal urethral closure pressure, and a history of previous incontinence treatment or prolapse repair, respectively. The procedure was successfully performed in all of the patients. Intra-operative complications included bladder injuries ($n = 5$, 0.8%), urethral injuries ($n = 2$, 0.3%), hemorrhage ($n = 3$, 0.5%) and vaginal perforation in ($n = 13$, 2.2%). There were no digestive, neurological or vascular complications. On four-hundred patients followed-up for at least 3 months, with a mean follow-up time of 11.7 months, 86.8% were cured, 7.7% improved and 5.5% failed.

Analysis of a sub-group of the French registry (25,26) has shown that the TOT is effective in association with prolapse repair (cure rates 80.6%, improvement 12.9%, failure 6.5%), in obese patients (cure rates 74.2%, improvement 9.7%, failure 16.1%), in recurrent urinary stress incontinence (cure rates 77.3%, improvement 9%, failure 13.7%), and in patients with intrinsic sphincter deficiency (cure rates 77.2%, improvement 9.1%, failure 13.7%).

Conclusions

The TOT technique is simple, quick, and safe. It allows accurate placement of a suburethral tape avoiding the pelvis. There have been no reports of vascular, digestive, or neurological complications. Vaginal, urethral, and bladder injuries may be avoided in most of the cases by close attention to the technical details previously described. Cystoscopy is not necessary in most patients. Use of a woven monofilament polypropylene tape is preferable to avoid vaginal wound healing defects and infection. Post-operative continence rates at one-year follow up is similar to the TVT procedure.

TRANSOBTURATOR VAGINAL TAPE INSIDE-OUT

Background

In 2003, J. de Leval modified the transobturator approach by reversing the direction by which the tape is inserted: from the suburethral incision to the skin incisions. This modification was called as the "inside-out transobturator vaginal tape" (TVT-O) by the author (27). The main objective of the modification was to further decrease the risk of bladder and urethral injuries associated with the TOT technique (21,24,28).

In order to determine the exact anatomical trajectory of the tape and its relationships with the neighboring neuro-vascular structures and organs, de Leval et al. have performed cadaver dissections (29). Seven female cadavers aged 65 years or more, with no history of prior pelvic or perineal intervention, were dissected. The positioning of the suburethral tape was carried out in each cadaver according to the standard operative protocol. The anterior perineal and obturator regions were thereafter dissected. The ischio-pubic ramus was sectioned and removed to ease the dissection. These studies demonstrated that the tape had followed the following consistent path: it penetrated from the suburethral space, at the junction between mid and distal urethra, into the anterior recess of the ischio-rectal fossa, limited medially and cranially by the levator ani muscle, caudally by the deep transverse muscle, and laterally by the internal obturator muscle. Then the tape perforated the obturator membrane and muscles and exited at the skin level after passing through the adductor muscles and sub-cutaneous tissues. The tape was at a significant distance from the terminal end of the pudendal nerve, which was located much more superficially; it was below the median perineal aponeurosis, the obturator nerve and vessels, and the femoral vessels. The obturator vascular structures were also carefully dissected. Dissections consistently showed that the anterior branch of the obturator artery lied on the external rim of the ischio-pubic ramus, and was thus protected by this bony structure from being injured by the insertion of the tape.

Like the TOT, the TVT-O tape passes from the perineal region through the obturator and thigh regions, without entering the pelvic cavity. The bladder, pudendal nerve and femoral and obturator neuro-vascular structures are distant from the tape's dissection track. The urethra and vaginal walls are under direct view.

Instrumentation

Special instruments have been produced to perform this procedure. The *"helical passers"* are a pair of instruments, specific for the left and right sides (Fig. 15). They are made of stainless steel comprising a spirally shaped section and a handle. The spiral section has an open circular segment of 3 cm radius terminated by two linear segments. On the horizontal plane perpendicular to the handle's axis, the gap between the extremities of the spiral section is 2 cm. The element supported by the helical passer is a hollow polyethylene "tube." It has a sharp pointed distal end (Fig. 15) and a lateral opening, which allows the insertion of the spiral segment of the helical passer into its lumen.

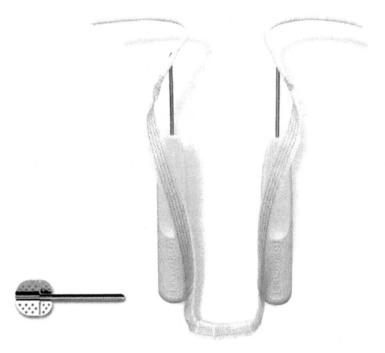

Figure 15 TVT-O inside-out instrumentation: helical passers, tubes, tape, and guide.

The third instrument is called the "guide." This is a stainless steel device that comprises a semi-circular gutter (Fig. 15). The guide acts both as a shoe-horn and as a lever arm to ease the slipping in of the passers, introduced alongside the gutter, from the perineal space through the obturator foramens. The guide also plays the role of a barrier, preventing the helical passer to enter the pelvic space. It permits to carry out a minimally invasive and reproducible dissection, which makes finger guidance unnecessary.

The TVT-O tape (Gynecare, Ethicon) is the same non-absorbable polypropylene tape as the one used in the TVT procedure, the only difference being its blue color (Fig. 15). The proximal end of the tube is opened and is attached to the tape together with its protective plastic sheath.

Surgical Technique

The procedure includes the following steps:

1. The patient is placed in the dorsal lithotomy position with the hips hyperflexed over the abdomen (±110°). The buttocks are positioned flush with the edge of the operating table.

2. The procedure can be carried out under local, regional or general anesthesia.
3. The operative field is prepared with a standard antiseptic agent and the patient draped, taking care to keep the groin folds in the operative field and the anus covered. Exposure of the vulvar vestibulum is enhanced by suturing the labia laterally.
4. An indwelling catheter is inserted into the bladder, which is emptied.
5. The exit points of the plastic tubes are marked with a felt pen, tracing a horizontal line at the level of the urethral meatus. A second line, that is parallel and 2 cm above the first is traced. It is on this line, 2 cm lateral to the folds of the thigh that the exit points will be located (Fig. 16). A 5-mm incision is made at each exit point.

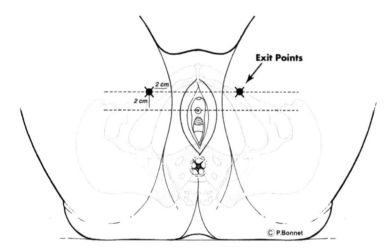

Figure 16 TVT-O inside-out surgical technique: Exit points are marked by tracing a horizontal line at the level of the urethral meatus, and a second line parallel and 2 cm above. Exit points are located on the second line, 2 cm lateral to the folds of the thigh.

6. Using Allis clamps for traction, a 1 cm midline incision is placed in the vaginal mucosa starting 1cm below the urethral meatus. Minimal paraurethral sub-mucosal dissection is then carried out laterally with a blade, over a few millimeters distance, on each side. It is recommended that insertion of the device be completed on one side before beginning the dissection of the contra lateral side. Using a "push-spread" technique, blunt dissection is carried out, preferably using pointed, curved scissors. The path of the lateral dissection must be orientated at

a 45° angle from the midline sagittal plane, with the tips of the scissors pointed slightly upward (Fig. 17). Dissection is continued toward the

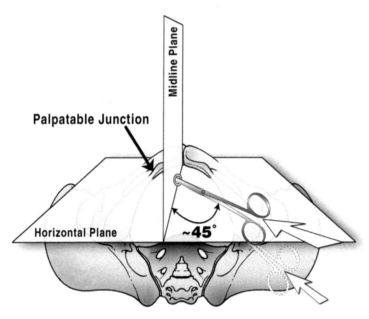

Figure 17 TVT-O inside-out surgical technique: Minimal para-urethral sub-vaginal dissection is carried out laterally using pointed and curved scissors. The lateral dissection should be orientated at a 45° angle from the midline sagittal plane, with the tips pointed slightly upward.

junction between the body of the pubic bone and the inferior pubic ramus. When the junction is reached, the tips of the scissors are pointed slightly downward to perforate the obturator membrane. A loss of resistance can be felt when the membrane is perforated. The channel should be approximately 5 to 7 mm in diameter and no deeper than 5 cm. If the bone is not reached after dissecting for 5 cm, it is essential to ascertain that the angle of dissection is correct.

7. The winged "guide" is inserted into the tract created, until it passes the ischio-pubic ramus and enters the opening previously made in the obturator membrane. Loss of resistance is felt as the winged guide passes through the obturator membrane. If difficulty is encountered during insertion of the guide, the direction of the tract should be reassessed with the scissors. The open side of the guide must be facing the operator. If necessary (e.g., in obese patients), the bendable tab may be bent to increase the length of the gutter of the guide from 6 to 7 cm.

8. The "helical passer" is inserted into the dissected tract following the channel of the winged guide. The device is pushed inward, traversing, and slightly passing the obturator membrane. At this point, it is important to orient the handle of the device in such a way that the straight tip of the helical passer is aligned with the channel in the winged guide and remains in that orientation until the tip reaches the obturator foramen (Fig. 18).

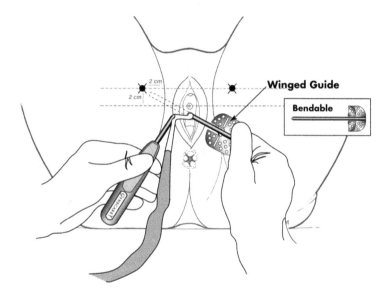

Figure 18   TVT-O inside-out surgical technique: Insertion of the helical passer into the dissected tract following the channel of the winged guide.

9. Once in this position, the winged guide is removed and kept sterile for later use on the other side.
10. Once the guide is removed, the handle of the helical passer is rotated (clockwise for patient's right side and counterclockwise for patient's left side) simultaneously as the handle is moved towards the midline (Fig. 19). The handle must never be orientated in a horizontal position.
11. The tip of the tube should exit near the previously determined exit points (Fig. 20). However, slight skin manipulation may be required. If the skin incision has not been previously made, it is now made where the tip of the helical passer tents the skin.
12. When the tip of the plastic tube appears at the skin opening, it is grasped with a clamp (Fig. 21) and, while stabilizing the tube near the urethra, the helical passer is removed by reverse rotation of the handle.

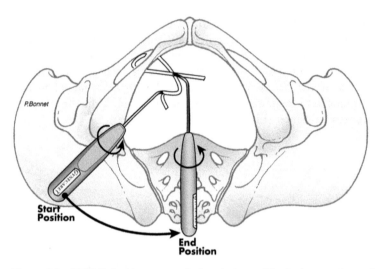

Figure 19 TVT-O inside-out surgical technique: Clockwise rotation of the helical passer on patient's right side.

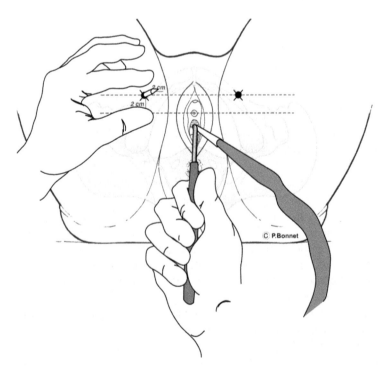

Figure 20 TVT-O inside-out surgical technique: Exit of the tip of the tube at the previously determined exit point.

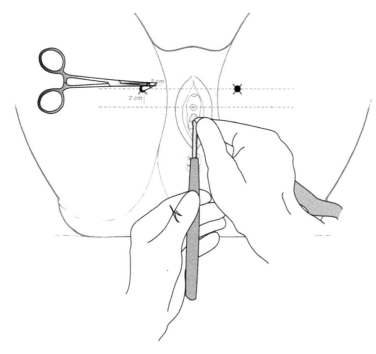

Figure 21   TVT-O inside-out surgical technique: Grasping of the plastic tube with a clamp when the tip appears at the exit point.

13. The plastic tube is pulled completely through the skin incision until the tape appears (Fig. 22).
14. The same procedure is repeated on the opposite side ensuring that the tape lies flat under the urethra (Fig. 23).
15. When both plastic tubes have been extracted through the skin incisions, the plastic tubes are cut off from the tape and plastic sheaths. The tape is positioned loosely, without tension, and flat under the urethra. At this stage a cough test may be performed. This allows adjustment of the tape so that only a few drops of urine are lost during the cough. When the tape is in position, the plastic sheaths that cover the tapes are removed (Fig. 24). As for the other procedures, to avoid positioning the tape with excess tension, a blunt instrument (e.g., scissors or forceps) is placed between the urethra and the tape during removal of the plastic sheaths, through the skin incisions.
16. Thereafter vaginal incision is closed. The tape ends are cut at the exit points just below the skin. The skin incisions are closed with suture or surgical adhesive tape.
17. Cystoscopy can be performed at the discretion of the surgeon. If cystoscopy was performed following the first passage, it is necessary to empty the bladder prior to initiating passage of the second side.

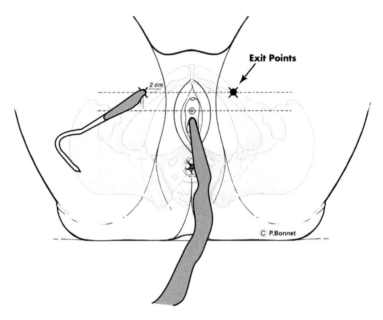

Figure 22 TVT-O inside-out surgical technique: The plastic tube is completely pulled through the skin until the tape appears.

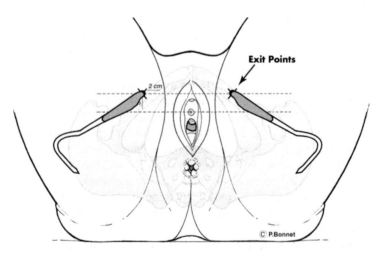

Figure 23 TVT-O inside-out surgical technique: The technique is repeated on the patient's other side ensuring that the tape lies flat under the urethra.

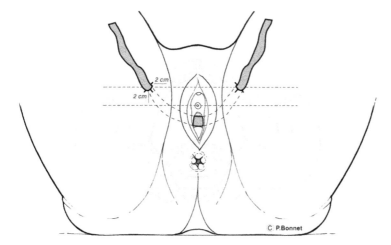

Figure 24   TVT-O inside-out surgical technique: Tape position under the urethra after extraction of both plastic tubes and removal of both plastic sheaths through the skin incisions.

Clinical Data

Since March 2002, de Leval et al. performed more than 375 TVT-O surgical procedures on patients who had clinically demonstrated urinary stress incontinence with a positive pre-operative cough stress test.

The initial feasibility study included 113 patients from March 2002 to March 2003 (27). In 77 patients, the TVT-O was the sole procedure and 36 had associated procedures for prolapse. The mean age of the patients was 62 years (range 29 to 88). The cohort of patients consisted of a hetero-geneous and unselected population since 30%, 10%, 44% and 15% of the subjects enrolled had pre-operative urgency incontinence, mixed incon-tinence, low maximal urethral closure pressure, and a history of previous incontinence or prolapse repair, respectively. All patients had a follow-up period of at least 6 months with a mean follow-up of 10 months. One patient was lost to follow-up at the one month visit, and 4 additional patients were lost to follow-up at the 6 months visit.

The procedure was successfully performed in all of the patients. All helical passers were passed through the obturator foramen and exited at the skin level exactly where it had been marked and incised. The mean operative time for the TVT-O procedure was 12 minutes (range 6–20). There were no urethral or bladder injuries and no significant bleeding during the procedure. There were no major post-operative complications such as obturator or thigh hematoma, neurological or bowel complica-tions, tape rejection or fistula. A minor vaginal wound healing defect was observed in one patient; this did not require further surgery. Urinary infection was noted in three patients. Superficial vein thrombosis occurred in one patient at day 8 after surgery, with secondary development of an abscess that required drainage; this abscess was located approximately 10 cm below the skin exit point of the passer. Nonetheless the outcome for the patient was favorable. After this adverse event, all patients were administered antibiotics prophylactically.

Among 108 patients with more than 6 months follow-up, 98 were cured (90.7%), 4 improved (3.7%) and 6 failed (5.6%). Urge symptoms disappeared or decreased in 72.8% and 6%, respectively, among the 33 patients who suffered from this condition pre-operatively. No change in urge symptoms was noted in five patients (15.2%) and six out of 96 patients developed de novo urge incontinence (6.25%). Seven patients (5.4%) experienced complete post-operative retention, which was treated medically in four patients and surgically in three patients, using an immediate tape release procedure.

Occurrence of pain was carefully recorded by the investigators. Seventeen patients (15%) described post-operative unilateral or bilateral pain. Pain was localized in the thighs ($n = 13$), hip region ($n = 2$), lumbar spine ($n = 1$) or was reported as sciatalgia ($n = 1$). Pain was always mild and limited to the first two post-operative days; none of the patients required opioid analgesics. Pain symptoms were not reported by any of the patients at the 1 month visit. Dyspareunia was reported by two patients at the 6 month visit.

A prospective study on 250 patients with short-term follow-up has confirmed these initial results (30). There were no urethra, bladder, digestive, neurological or vaginal complications. Results showed a complete cure rate of urinary stress incontinence of 94%.

Conclusions

The inside-out TVT-O technique is simple, quick, and safe. It allows the accurate passage of the tape with minimal dissection, protection of the urethra and avoiding the pelvis. There have been no reported urethra or bladder injuries and no vascular, digestive or neurological complications. Cystoscopy is normally not necessary. Post-operative continence rates are similar to the TVT procedure on short-term follow-up.

SUMMARY AND CONCLUSIONS

Three surgical procedures that are based on the placement of a synthetic suburethral sling are now available for treatment of USI. The TVT is an effective, minimally invasive surgical technique, with 10 years of follow-up, that yield cure and improvement rates comparable to more invasive approaches, such as the Burch procedure performed via laparotomy or laparoscopy. However, due to the intra- or post-operative complications referred to in the text, we believe that the transobturator route is preferable to the TVT.

The transobturator route is performed in two ways: the out-inside and inside-out approach. Both of these approaches are simple, quick, safe and do not require routine cystoscopy. The para-urethral subvaginal dissection is less extensive with the inside-out route and the learning curve of this approach appears to be quicker for residents. However, it would be desirable for each surgeon to attempt both techniques in order to determine which of the two they prefer.

REFERENCES

1. Ulmsten U, Petros P. Intravaginal slingplasty: an ambulatory surgical procedure for treatment of female incontinence. Scand J Urol Nephrol 1995; 29:75–82.
2. Ulmsten U, Johnson P, Rezapour M. A three-year follow-up of tension free vaginal tape for surgical treatment of female urinary stress incontinence. Br J Obstet Gynaecol 1999; 106:345–50.
3. Olsson I, Kroon U. A three-year postoperative evaluation of tension-free vaginal tape. Gynecol Obstet Invest 1999; 48:267–9.
4. Nilsson CG, Rezapour M, Falconer C et al. Seven years follow-up of the tension-free vaginal tape (TVT) procedure. Int Urogynecol J Pelvic Floor Dysfunct 2003; 14(Suppl 1):S35.
5. Delorme E. Transobturator urethral suspension: mini-invasive procedure in the treatment of urinary stress incontinence in women. Prog Urol 2001; 11:1306–13. (French).
6. Rezapour M, Ulmsten U. Tension-Free Vaginal Tape in women with mixed urinary incontinence: a long-term follow-up. Int Urogynecol J Pelvic Floor Dysfunct 2001; Suppl 2:S15–18.
7. Rezapour M, Ulmsten U. Tension-Free Vaginal Tape in women with recurrent urinary stress incontinence: a long-term follow-up. Int Urogynecol J Pelvic Floor Dysfunct 2001; Suppl 2:S9–11.
8. Rezapour M, Falconer C, Ulmsten U. Tension-Free Vaginal Tape in women with intrinsic sphincter deficiency: a long-term follow-up. Int Urogynecol J Pelvic Floor Dysfunct 2001; Suppl 2:S12–14.
9. Ward KL, Hilton P; UK and Ireland TVT Trial Group. A prospective multicenter randomized trial of tension-free vaginal tape and colposuspension for primary urodynamic stress incontinence: two-year follow-up. Am J Obstet Gynecol 2004; 190(2):324–31.
10. Maher C, Qatawneh A, Baessler K, Cropper M, Schluter P. Laparoscopic colposuspension or tension-free vaginal tape for recurrent urinary stress incontinence and/or intrinsic sphincter deficiency: a randomised controlled trial. Neurourol Urodynamics 2004; 23(5/6):433–4 (Abstract).

11. Wiskind AK, Creighton SM, Stanton SL. The incidence of genital prolapse after Burch colposuspension. Am J Obstet Gynecol 1992; 167:399–405.
12. Peyrat L, Boutin JM, Bruyere F, Haillot O, Fakfak H, Lanson Y. Intestinal perforation as a complication of tension-free vaginal tape procedure for urinary incontinence. Eur Urol 2001; 39(5):603–5.
13. Vierhout ME. Severe hemorrhage complicating tension-free vaginal tape: a case report. Int Urogynecol J Pelvic Floor Dysfunct 2001; 12(2):139–40.
14. Lim YN, Rane A, Barry C, Corstiaans A, Dietz HP, Muller R. The suburethral slingplasty evaluation study in North Qeensland (Suspend): a randomized controlled trial. Neurourol Urodynamics 2004; 23(5/6):495–6 (Abstract).
15. Soulie M, Cuvillier X, Benaissa A, Mouly P, Larroque JM, Bernstein J et al. The tension-free transvaginal tape procedure in the treatment of female urinary stress incontinence: a French prospective multicentre study. Eur Urol 2001; 39: 709–14 (Discussion 715).
16. Boustead GB. The Tension-free vaginal tape for treating female urinary stress incontinence. BJU Int 2002; 89:687–93.
17. Pifarotti P, Meschia M, Gattei U, Bernasconi F, Magatti F, Vignano R. Multicenter randomized trial of TVT and IVS for the treatment of urinary stress incontinence in Women. Neurourol Urodynamics 2004; 23(5/6):494–5 (Abstract).
18. Dargent D, Bretones S, George P, Mellier G. Insertion of a suburethral sling through the obturator membrane in the treatment of female urinary incontinence. Gynecol Obstet Fertil 2002; 30:576 (French).
19. Delorme E, Droupy S, de Tayrac R, Delmas V. Transobturator tape (Uratape): a new minimally-invasive procedure to treat female urinary incontinence. Eur Urol 2004; 45:2–203.
20. Costa P, Grise P, Droupy S et al. Surgical treatment of female urinary stress incontinence with a Trans-Obturator Tape (T.O.T.) Uratape: short term results of a prospective multicentric study. Eur Urol 2004; 46:1–102.
21. Game X, Mouzin M, Vaessen C, Malavaud B, Sarramon JP, Rischmann P. Obturator infected hematoma and urethral erosion following transoburator tape implantation. J Urol 2004; 171(4):1629.
22. Cindolo L, Salzano L, Rota G, Bellini S, D'Afiero A. Tension-free transobturator approach for female urinary stress incontinence. Minerva Urol Nefrol 2004; 56:1–89.
23. Mellier G, Benayed B, Bretones S, Pasquier JC. Suburethral tape via the obturator route: is the TOT a simplification of the TVT? Int Urogynecol J Pelvic Floor Dysfunct 2004; 15:4–227.
24. Hermieu JF. Trans-obturator tape for the treatment of female urinary stress incontinence: a multicentric prospective study. Presented at the annual meeting of the Association Française d'Urology, Paris, 2004.
25. Costa P. TOT multicenter register: results in specific subgroups (recurrent incontinence and low urethral closure pressure). Presented at the annual meeting of the International Continence Society & International Urogynecology Association, Paris, 2004.
26. de Tayrac R. TOT multicenter register: results in specific subgroups (associated prolapse and obese patients). Presented at the annual meeting of

the International Continence Society & International Urogynecology Association, Paris, 2004.

27. de Leval J. Novel surgical technique for the treatment of female urinary stress incontinence: transobturator vaginal tape inside-out. Eur Urol 2003; 44:724.
28. Minaglia S, Ozel B, Klutke C, Ballard C, Klutke J. Bladder injury during transobturator sling. Urology 2004; 64:376.
29. Bonnet P, Waltregny D, Reul O, de Leval J. Inside-out transobturator approach for the surgical treatment of female urinary stress incontinence: Anatomical considerations. Presented at the annual meeting of the European Association of Urology, Vienna, 2004.
30. Waltregny D, Reul O, Bonnet P, de Leval J. Inside-out transobturator vaginal tape (TVT-O): Short-term results of a prospective study. Presented at the annual meeting of the International Continence Society & International Urogynecology Association, Paris, 2004.

7

Evidence-Based Medicine on the Surgical Treatment of Urinary Stress Incontinence and Genital Prolapse

Hervé Fernandez

Service de Gynécologie-Obstétrique et d'Histologie-Embryologie-Cytogénétique à orientation Biologique et Génétique de la Reproduction, Hôpital Antoine Béclère, Assistance Publique-Hôpitaux de Paris, Clamart, France

Renaud de Tayrac

Groupe Hospitalier Caremeau, Service de Gynécologie-Obstétrique du Pr Mares, Nîmes, France

INTRODUCTION

In order for those who practice medicine to keep current, it is essential to interpret and criticize the results of clinical investigations of new techniques before integrating them to practice.

Evidence-based medicine is the conscientious, explicit, and judicious use of the best evidence to determine the effectiveness and safety of therapeutic interventions. Developments in information technology and the Internet have assisted the introduction of evidence-based medicine into our practice.

Evidence-based medicine is comprised of five steps:

1. Setting a clinical question
2. Finding the best evidence
3. Appraising the evidence
4. Integrating the evidence
5. Auditing clinical practice

These steps of research evidence allow professionals to categorize studies as either primary (randomized control trial, cohort, case control, cross-sectional or case series) or secondary (systematic review with or without meta-analysis, guidelines).

The rationale of the surgical treatment of urinary stress incontinence (USI) and genital prolapse has changed over the past few years because of the introduction of techniques of urethral suspension that use slings and the surgical management of urogenital prolapse by vaginal approach with the use of meshes. These new surgical approaches need to be assessed based on evidence before they are incorporated into the therapeutic strategy. Figure 1 summarizes the concept of evaluation for a new operation.

URINARY INCONTINENCE

Urinary incontinence is a common problem throughout the world, although it is not always confessed. USI as recently defined by the International Continence Society (1), is the complaint of involuntary leakage of urine during effort or exertion or during sneezing or coughing. More than 200 operative procedures have been described for the treatment of USI. Many of these are modifications of the same procedure; but there is not one single definitive operation. Surgery is recommended if conservative treatment fails i.e. cure rates of around 50% have been reported with physiotherapy (2).

Open colposuspension (Burch procedure) has been regarded as the gold standard for operative treatment of USI (3). Laparoscopic approaches were introduced in the beginning of the 1990s. Vancaillie and Schuessler (4) were the first to describe a laparoscopic technique for bladder neck suspension. Modifications were published later, using mesh or surgical staples, including an extra peritoneal approach.

Ankardal et al. (5) performed randomized clinical trials (RCT) comparing open Burch colposuspension ($n = 120$) with laparoscopic colposuspension using mesh and staples ($n = 120$). Open colposuspension had higher objective and subjective cure rates one year after surgery, but was associated

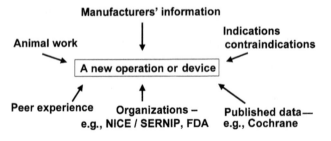

Figure 1   Evidence-based medicine and urogynecology.

with greater blood loss, greater risk of urinary retention, and a longer hospital stay; all issues that must be included in the equation.

The midurethral concept concerning the mechanisms of female USI was presented in 1990 by Petros and Ulmsten (6). Based on this new theory, the tension-free vaginal tape (TVT) procedure was developed for its surgical treatment.

This procedure, which is simple, safe, effective and speedy has revolutionized the surgical treatment of USI and has popularized minimally invasive approaches. Since its first description, many other mid-urethral tapes have been incorporated into clinical practice, unfortunately without prior animal and controlled clinical trials for most of these.

Many of the reports written about these new devices are short series with inadequate statistics and always a short follow-up. Therefore, we need to be rigorous in the selection of studies and we must include only the studies with sufficient numbers of patients, statistical power, and standardized criteria and a minimum follow-up of two years.

Nilsson et al. (7) has reported the long-term cure rates and late complications rates after seven-year follow-up of the TVT procedure for treatment of USI. Eighty out of 90 women were available for follow-up. Both objective and subjective cure rates were 81.3% with de novo urge symptoms in 6.3%. No signs of tape erosion or any tissue reactions indicating tape material rejection were found. This absence of long-term adverse events associated with a high subjective and objective cure rates make the TVT operation a recommendable surgical treatment for female USI, and confirm that TVT is the new gold standard surgery for USI treatment.

Due to these satisfactory outcomes with the TVT procedure, RCT were performed between TVT and colposuspension techniques, which was the most popular choice for primary surgery with reported cure rates of up to 96% (8). Ward and Hilton (9) have reported the 2-year follow-up of 344 women in a RCT comparing TVT and open Burch colposuspension. The objective cure rates defined as a negative 1-hour pad test, ranged from 63% to 85% for the TVT procedure and 51% to 87% for open colposuspension. Subjectively, only 43% of patients in the TVT group and 37% in the open colposuspension group reported cure of their stress leakage. These results are similar to those reported by Black et al. (10), in their large cohort study. The success rate reported in this trial is lower than most published series for USI surgery. However, most studies report success rate based on a poorly defined population with non validated outcome measures.

Many RCTs, Table 1 (9,11–15) compared TVT with colposuspension, which has been the gold standard for the treatment of USI. As evident from Table 1, the results of TVT and colposuspension are fairly similar.

However, it is also necessary to assess the proportion of de novo urge incontinence and overactive bladder symptoms after TVT. Segal et al. (16) demonstrated that 57% of patients with preoperative overactive bladder symptoms can expect resolution of these symptoms after a TVT. The

Table 1 TVT/Burch: Results of Randomized Clinical Trial

	Ward 2004 (9)	Valpas 2004 (11)	Paraiso 2004 (12)	Ustun 2003 (13)	Liang 2002 (14)	Liapis 2002 (15)
TVT (n)	175	70	36	23	23	36
Burch (n)	169 (open)	51 (laparoscopic)	36 (laparoscopic)	23 (laparoscopic)	22	35
Objective success rate % for TVT	63	85.7	96.8	82.6	82.6	84
Objective success rate % for Burch	51	56.9	81.2	82.6	77.3	86
Month follow-up	24	12	20.6	3	20	24
95% CI or P	<0.01	12.7–43.9	P<0.05	NS	NS	NS

Abbreviations: CI, confidence interval; TVT, tension-free vaginal tape.

proportion of patients in whom de novo overactive bladder (4.3%) and de novo urge incontinence (9.1%) symptoms developed post operatively is low.

The most common intra-operative complications with TVT include bladder injury at the time of trocar insertion and bleeding in the retropubic space. In response to the concern that the retropubic passage of a trocar carried with it the potential complication of bladder or vascular and urethral injury, Delorme (17) has described a transobturator tape (TOT, Mentor-Porgès) that passed horizontally by an out-inside approach under the urethra and was less likely to injure it. Since, many other modifications of this new technique have already been introduced.

A new TVT-O procedure (Gynecare, Ethicon) using an inside-out approach to minimize urethral and bladder injury has been proposed (18). But, at this time, there is no objective evidence that it is any safer than the out-inside type sling procedure. There have been few RCTs with these new surgical approaches. Arunkalaivanan and Barrington (19) compared TVT ($n = 68$) with pelvicol sling ($n = 74$) with a 12 months follow-up. The success rate was respectively 85% and 89% (NS).

Neuman (20) compared two anti-incontinence operations: the TVT and the TVT-O for the first two 75 patients groups. In this studies, the TVT-obturator patients seem to have less intra-operative and post-operative surgical complications than the TVT patients with the same early therapeutic failure rates, respectively 1.3% and 2.7% with one year follow-up.

Another RCT (21) compared the retropubic (RPR) approach (42 cases) with a transobturator route (TOR) out-inside (46 cases). The immediate functional results were similar. The suburethral sling procedure was less painful by the TOR route than by the RPR route. Bladder injury, hematomas and abscesses were only observed in RPR group, while vaginal injury only occurred in the TOR group.

Two other RCTs have been published. Vervest et al. (23) compared TVT-O® ($n = 39$) and MonarC® ($n = 36$) i.e., In-out versus out-in. The effectiveness was similar but one vaginal perforation occurred with the out-in route. Wang et al. (22) compared Monarc® versus Sparc® i.e., out-in transobturator suburethral sling versus suprapubic sling procedure. The out-in route appeared more painful (12.9 % vs 0 %) with a trend to vaginal perforation (12.9 % *vs.* 0 %).

The last RCT (24) reported the same success rate between the classic TVT method and TVT-O, with 12 months follow-up. This result is interesting because it tested the same sling with both routes. However, all these comparative or randomized trials have a short follow-up evaluation.

In conclusion, sub-urethral slings are becoming the gold standard of surgical treatment for USI but some questions remain: The choice between retro-pubic or transobturator approach and in transobturator approach the choice between out-in and in-out insertion. In the first instance functional results are similar. Intraoperative cystoscopy is not mandatory with the transobturator approaches. The current trend appears to favor the trans-obturator approach, because it is safer, quicker, and easier to learn.

Nonetheless, the scientific answer will require RCTs with appropriate number of patients, statistics, and suitable subjective and objective outcomes, after a minimum follow-up period of over 2 years and long-term evaluation of erosion and voiding difficulties.

GENITAL PROLAPSE

The incidence of pelvic organ prolapse increases with age, and the proportion of population increases along with the progresses in medicine. The lifetime risk of surgery for prolapse by age 80 years is estimated to be 11.1% (25).

The main goal of surgical treatment is to correct the anatomical defect(s) and functional troubles and to preserve vaginal function. The existence of many surgical techniques demonstrates the absence of a gold standard method, and the pelvic surgeon is faced with a dilemma when selecting the most appropriate procedure. Moreover, the rates of recurrence remain high, up to 30%.

There are three ways of access in reconstructive pelvic surgery (abdominal laparoscopic and vaginal) for the repair of anterior (cystocele), median (hysterocele, vaginal vault), and posterior (rectocele) defects. The choice often depends exclusively on the surgeon's experience.

The abdominal approach with sacrocolpopexy with use of mesh is considered the gold standard. The laparoscopic approach provides a similar outcome. The drawback of this approach remains laparoscopic suturing. The vaginal approach was reserved classically for older women but the use of biological or synthetic meshes have modified indications during the last few years.

The conventional surgical procedures of anterior and posterior colporrhaphy associated with repair of bilateral transvaginal and paravaginal defects, together with sacrospinous ligament fixation, are associated with a recurrence rate of 20% to 50% (26–28). This rate of recurrence clearly demonstrates the need to improve these techniques. The use of a synthetic mesh in vaginal surgery was first introduced by Julian (29). The placement of a mesh aims at reducing the recurrence rate and preventing stenosis and dyspareunia. The rate of complications with meshes, non-absorbable, composite or absorbable (including vaginal erosions, formation of a sinus trajectory, prosthesis ablation, urethral erosion), beg the question: "which mesh should be used?"

The Meshes

Completely absorbable materials (Dexon® and Vicryl®) have no place in the repair of pelvic defects. Manufactured non-absorbable materials are based on polypropylene: Prolene® (Ethicon), Marlex® (Bard), Gynemesh® (Gynecare,

Ethicon), Soft prolene® (Gynecare, Ethicon), Pelvitex® (Sofradim & Bard), or polyethylene-tèrephtalate: Mersuture® (Ethicon), Parietex® (Sofradim). These meshes have varying weight/m², thickness, porosity, and spaces (Table 2).

The type of incision can influence the rate of erosions; with the use of sagittal colpotomies on the anterior and posterior vaginal walls, a 19.5% erosion rate has been observed with Prolene® standard mesh, whereas with the use of transverse colpotomy and Prolene soft® mesh, the erosion rate was only 3.3% (30). This significant decrease in erosion can be attributed to the absence of scar facing the mesh and the use of mesh with largest spaces (Table 3). Moreover, the absence of hysterectomy decreased the erosion rate.

Treatment of Anterior Prolapse

Anterior colporrhaphy is recommended for central defects with plication of the vesicopelvic fasciae and bladder neck. Anterior repair has been the gold standard for cystocele repair (31). The recurrence rate varies from 3% to 22% at a mean follow-up of 2 to 20 years (31–34).

In case of lateral defects, paravaginal repair is recommended. The paravaginal defects are repaired using permanent suture incorporating the pubocervical fascia, the arcus tendineous, and the vaginal wall. The pelvic side wall can be accessed vaginally or laparoscopically (35,36). However, frequent complications and technical difficulty with the vaginal approach to paravaginal repair has limited its widespread use in clinical practice.

To decrease recurrence rate, prosthetic reinforcement has been employed for anterior colporrhaphy. In a RCT, Sand et al. (37) treated 80 patients with absorbable mesh (Polyglactin 910) and 80 without. At 1-year follow-up, 43% of those in whom mesh was not used and 25% of those who had mesh had recurrent cystoceles. In another RCT, use of absorbable mesh was more effective than the standard anterior colporraphy alone (38).

Table 2 Comparative Wand Thickness of the Different Synthetic Meshes

Brand	Weight (g/m²)	Thickness (mm)	Porosity (%)	Largest space (mm)
Surgipro 1	84	0.38		
Surgipro 2	103.6	0.46	35	
Surgipro 3	97.6	0.59	50	
Gynemesh	96.6	0.64	50	0.7
New Prolene	77	0.53		
Gynemesh soft	42.7	0.42	64	2.4
Pelvitex	38	0.4	89	1.5

Table 3   Erosion Phenomenon

TVM		n	Erosion	%
With sagittal colpotomy	Prolene mesh	56	11	19.6
	Prolene soft	7	0	0
With transversal colpotomy	Prolene mesh	4	0	0
	Prolene soft	33	1	3.3

Source: From Ref. 30.

The use of non-absorbable mesh is becoming a promising option. But based on experience to date it is preferable to use the nonwoven poly-propylene monofilament mesh because of its effectiveness. A RCT has shown, at 2-year follow-up, a reduced rate of recurrence with the Marlex mesh (28). Many other prospective and retrospective nonrandomized studies have reported high success rates, ranging from 75% to 100%, at short and median-term follow-up (Table 4). However, there was still a relatively high vaginal erosion rate (49). This is also encountered with abdominal prolapse repair when hysterectomy performed in the same time.

Vaginal Vault Prolapse

The incidence of vaginal vault prolapse has been estimated to occur in 0.1% to 4.5% after hysterectomy whatever the surgical access used (52,53). The most common procedure for the treatment of vault prolapse is abdominal sacrocolpopexy, using several types of synthetic material. Lefranc et al. (54) has reported experience with a median follow-up of 10.5 years and only 2.3% relapse. The morbidity of this technique is osteomyelitis and mesh erosion (2.7–9%). The combined abdominal-vaginal approach increased the incidence of mesh erosion for 3.2% to 40%.

Mesh erosion into the bladder or into the rectum or the vagina occurred in approximately 5% of patients and constituted about 50% of the complications requiring reoperation.

Laparoscopic sacrocolpopexy was first described by Nezhat et al. (55). The advantages of this approach over the abdominal are due to the better visualization of the operative field that permits safe dissection and accurate suture placement.

Cosson et al. (56) have reported 93% satisfaction rate with good anatomical results in a retrospective study. However, the degree of technical difficulty of this technique has limited its widespread acceptance.

Vaginal approach of the vaginal vault prolapse has been popularized by Randall and Nichols in United States (57) and Richter in Europe. Vaginal vault suspension to the sacrospinous ligaments can be done uni-laterally or bilaterally. However, there have been no RCT to compare the two types of fixations. Subjective or objective cure rates of 77% to 82%

Table 4 Literature Series of Transvaginal Cystocele Repair with Synthetic Meshes

Author	Year	Mesh	n	Follow-up (months)	Anatomical success rate (%)	Vaginal infection (%)	Vaginal erosion (%)
Julian (29)	1996	Marlex	12	24	100	0	8.3
Nicita (39)	1998	Marlex	44	3	93.2	0	2.3
Flood (40)	1998	Marlex	142	36	94.4	3.5	2.1
Mage (41)	1999	Mersuture	46	26	100	0	2.2
Migliari (42)	2000	Prolene	12	20	75	0	0
Hardiman (43)	2000	GyneMesh	18	1	100	0	11.1
Eglin (44)	2003	Pelvitex	103	18	97	0	5
Sergent (45)	2003	Prolene	26	6	100	0	0
Adhoute (46)	2004	GyneMesh	52	27	95	0	3.8
Shah (47)	2004	Prolene	29	25	93.3	0	6.7
Dwyer (48)	2004	Atrium	47	29	94	0	7
Milani (49)	2004	Prolene	63	17	94	0	13
de Tayrac (50)	2005	GyneMesh	87	24	91.6	0	8.3
Total			681		94.4 (75–100)	0.27 (0–3.5)	5.4 (0–13)

have been reported with this technique along with an incidence of 3% of gluteal pain, which usually resolves spontaneously within 6 months (58). Posterior intravaginal sling plasty is a new procedure for the treatment of vault prolapse. A RCT with the Richter procedure has been commenced in our center.

Treatment of Posterior Compartment

Large rectoceles may cause symptoms such as incomplete bowel emptying, vaginal mass, and pressure. Numerous techniques have also been described for the surgical repair of rectocele. Ho et al. (59) proposed a transanal approach but it compromised anal sphincter pressures with a risk of impaired anal sphincter function.

The recurrence rate at one-year follow-up after posterior colporrhaphy or site-specific posterior colporrhaphy has been reported as 18% to 24% (60–62). This rate of recurrence induced the use of prosthetic material. Sand et al. (37) in a prospective RCT comparing the efficacy of posterior colporrhaphy with or without polyglactin 910 mesh have shown no difference between the two groups, with a 24% recurrence rate. Outcomes of use of non-absorbable meshes is available only from observational studies (63–65) summarized in Table 5. Although these report better results, a longer follow-up period is necessary to confirm the absence of recurrence and the risk of erosion and to evaluate coital function.

Can RCTs shed light on what is the best approach? There have been only three prospective randomized controlled trials reported between abdominal and vaginal approaches. The first one was by Benson et al. (28); they compared vaginal sacrospinous vault suspension ($n = 48$) versus abdominal sacrocolpopexy ($n = 40$). The median follow-up was 2.5 years (1–5.5). The patients operated by the vaginal route had a greater rate of recurrence of cystocele (29% vs. 10%), vaginal vault prolapse (12% vs. 3%), and dyspareunia (15% vs. 5%). Two other RCTs have been published in 2004. Maher et al. (66) compared vaginal sacrospinous vault suspension

Table 5 Literature Series of Transvaginal Rectocele Repair with Synthetic Meshes

Author	Year	*n*	Follow-up (months)	Mesh	Cure rate (%)	Erosion rate (%)
Watson (63)	1996	9	29	Marlex	89	
Sullivan (64)	2001	90	60	Marlex	100	5
Von Theobald (65)	2003	92	12	Surgipro	99	3.3
Totals					96	4

($n = 48$) and abdominal sacrocolpopexy ($n = 47$) for vaginal vault prolapse after hysterectomy. There was no difference between the two groups for subjective and objective results.

Roovers et al. (67) performed a global RCT comparing abdominal and vaginal prolapse surgery. They found that vaginal hysterectomy with anterior and/or posterior colporraphy was preferable to abdominal sacrocolpopexy with preservation of the uterus in surgical correction of uterine prolpase stages II-IV. The rate of re-operation was 1 of the 41 for patients who underwent vaginal surgery and 9 of the 41 after abdominal surgery. This greater rate of reoperation after abdominal surgery, which is considered the gold standard, is surprising. Therefore a final conclusion is impossible in the absence of studies with significant power and a true definition of the end-point (recurrence and sexual activity).

Women with severe genital prolapse may also have clinical urinary stress incontinence, but often they are continent subjectively because of urethral kinking or compression. Reduction of the prolapse as a result of surgery may reveal occult USI. Meschia et al. as a result of a RCT recommended use of TVT to decrease the incidence of post-operative USI (68). In a retrospective case-control study (69), we reported that, in patient with genital prolapse and USI, TVT was more effective than prosthetic cystocele repair alone to prevent postoperative USI; there was no difference in voiding dysfunction. Conversely in patients with occult USI, prosthetic cystocele repair was as effective as TVT.

The last question to address is the consequence of USI surgery and/or pelvic organ prolapse surgery about social, physiologic, occupational, domestic, physical and sexual well-being of women. Rogers (70) assessed the sexual function with the pelvic organ prolapse urinary incontinence sexual questionnaire (PISQ). The study showed the absence of improvement in sexual function, pronounced in women who underwent concomitant prolapse surgery and despite improvement of incontinence 3 to 6 months after surgery. Postoperative counselling may play an important role in returning women to their preoperative level of function.

CONCLUSION

USI is a common and troublesome problem for women. The Burch colposuspension has been considered as the gold standard, as a result of long-term objective incontinence cure rates.

Since 1996, when TVT was first described for correction of USI, the procedure has been used extensively. It yields high success rates, and the RCTs confirmed the equivalence of success rates with Burch colposuspension and with less morbidity. In 2001, the transobturator vaginal tape was introduced, using either the out-in or the in-out approach for the placement of the tape. The TOR is appealing because of its simplicity, safety, and the lower risk of bladder perforation. The RCTs showed no difference in outcomes between out-in and in-out approaches. Experience showed a shorter learning curve with the in-out route, due to a shorter medium sagittal incision of the vaginal wall and the insertion of winged guide.

In regard to treatment of pelvic organ prolapse, RCTs do not provide clear conclusions. Three RCTs reported no difference.between abdominal and vaginal approaches. The use of meshes increased the success rate of the vaginal approach but the rate of mesh erosion and shrinkage could limit further development of these techniques. Studies must be undertaken to evaluate sexual function following surgical treatment of pelvic organ prolapse with both abdominal and vaginal approaches.

REFERENCES

1. Abrams P, Cardozo L, Fall M, et al. Standardisation Sub-committee of the International Continence Society. The standardisation of terminology of lower urinary tract function: report from the Standardisation Sub-committee of the International Continence Society. Neurourol Urodyn 2002; 21(2):167–78.
2. Bo K, Talseth T, Holme I. Single blind, randomised controlled trial of pelvic floor exercises, electrical stimulation, vaginal cones, and no treatment in management of genuine stress incontinence in women. BMJ. 1999; 318(7182): 487–93.
3. Bidmead J, Cardozo L. Retropubic urethropexy (Burch colposuspension). Int Urogynecol J Pelvic Floor Dysfunct 2001; 12(4):262–5.
4. Vancaillie TG, Schuessler W. Laparoscopic bladderneck suspension. J Laparoendosc Surg 1991; 1(3):169–73.
5. Ankardal M, Ekerydh A, Crafoord K, Milsom I, Stjerndahl JH, Engh ME. A randomised trial comparing open Burch colposuspension using sutures with laparoscopic colposuspension using mesh and staples in women with urinary stress incontinence. BJOG 2004; 111(9):974–81.
6. Petros PE, Ulmsten UI. An integral theory of female urinary incontinence. Experimental and clinical considerations. Acta Obstet Gynecol Scand Suppl 1990; 153:7–31.
7. Nilsson CG, Falconer C, Rezapour M. Seven-year follow-up of the tension-free vaginal tape procedure for treatment of urinary incontinence. Obstet Gynecol 2004; 104(6):1259–62.
8. Jarvis GJ. Surgery for genuine stress incontinence. Br J Obstet Gynaecol 1994; 101(5):371–4.
9. Ward KL, Hilton P; UK and Ireland TVT Trial Group. A prospective multicenter randomized trial of tension-free vaginal tape and colposuspension for primary urodynamic stress incontinence: two-year follow-up. Am J Obstet Gynecol 2004; 190(2):324–31.
10. Black N, Griffiths J, Pope C, Bowling A, Abel P. Impact of surgery for stress incontinence on morbidity: cohort study. BMJ 1997; 315(7121):1493–8.

11. Valpas A, Kivela A, Penttinen J, Kujansuu E, Haarala M, Nilsson CG. Tension-free vaginal tape and laparoscopic mesh colposuspension for urinary stress incontinence. Obstet Gynecol 2004; 104(1):42–9.

12. Paraiso MF, Walters MD, Karram MM, Barber MD. Laparoscopic Burch colposuspension versus tension-free vaginal tape: a randomized trial. Obstet Gynecol 2004; 104(6):1249–58.

13. Ustun Y, Engin-Ustun Y, Gungor M, Tezcan S. Tension-free vaginal tape compared with laparoscopic Burch urethropexy. (Erratum in: J Am Assoc Gynecol Laparosc 2003; 10(4):581.) J Am Assoc Gynecol Laparosc 2003; 10(3):386–9.

14. Liang CC, Soong YK. Tension-free vaginal tape versus laparoscopic bladder neck suspension for urinary stress incontinence. Chang Gung Med J 2002; 25(6):360–6.

15. Liapis A, Bakas P, Creatsas G. Burch colposuspension and tension-free vaginal tape in the management of urinary stress incontinence in women. Eur Urol 2002; 41(4):469–73.

16. Segal JL, Vassallo B, Kleeman S, Silva WA, Karram MM. Prevalence of persistent and de novo overactive bladder symptoms after the tension-free vaginal tape. Obstet Gynecol 2004; 104(6):1263–9.

17. Delorme E. Transobturator urethral suspension: mini-invasive procedure in the treatment of urinary stress incontinence in women. Prog Urol 2001; 11(6): 1306–13.

18. De Leval J. Novel surgical technique for the treatment of female urinary stress incontinence: transobturator vaginal tape inside-out. Eur Urol 2003; 44(6): 724–30.

19. Arunkalaivanan AS, Barrington JW. Randomized trial of porcine dermal sling (Pelvicol implant) vs. tension-free vaginal tape (TVT) in the surgical treatment of stress incontinence: a questionnaire-based study. Int Urogynecol J Pelvic Floor Dysfunct 2003; 14(1):17–23 (Discussion 21—2).

20. Neuman M. TVT and TVT-Obturator: Comparison of two operative procedures. Eur J Obstet Gynecol Reprod Biol 2006; (Epub ahead of print).

21. David-Montefiore E, Frobert J-L, Grisard-Anaf M, et al. Peri-operative complications and pain after the suburethral sling procedure for urinary stress incontinence: a French prospective randomised multicentre study comparing the retropubic and transobturator routes. Eur Urol 2006; 49:133–8.

22. Wang AC, Lin YH, Tseng LH, Chih SY, Lee CJ. Prospective randomized comparison of transobturator suburethral sling (Monarc) vs suprapubic arc (Sparc) sling procedures for female urodynamic stress incontinence. Int Urogynecol J Pelvic Floor Dysfunct 2005; 3:1–5.

23. Vervest HAM, Bruin JP, Renes-Zeijl CC. Transobturator tape, inside-out or outside-in approaches: does it matter? Int Urogynecol J Pelvic Floor Dysfunct 2005; 16:S69.

24. Liapis A, Bakas P, Giner M, Creatsas G. Tension-free vaginal tape versus tension-free vaginal tape obturator in women with urinary stress incontinence. Gynecol Obstet Invest 2006 16; 62(3):160–4.

25. Olsen AL, Smith VJ, Bergstrom JO, Colling JC, Clark AL. Epidemiology of surgically managed pelvic organ prolapse and urinary incontinence. Obstet Gynecol 1997; 89(4):501–6.

26. Miyazaki FS, Miyazaki DW. Raz four-corner suspension for severe cystocele: poor results. Int Urogynecol J 1994; 5:94–7.

27. Kohli N, Sze EHM, Roat TW, Karram MM. Incidence of recurrent cystocele after anterior colporrhaphy with or without concomitant transvaginal needle suspension. Am J Obstet Gynecol 1996; 175:1476–82.

28. Benson J, Lucente V, McClellan E. Vaginal versus abdominal reconstructive surgery for the treatment of pelvic support defects: a prospective randomized study with long-term outcome evaluation. Am J Obstet Gynecol 1996; 175: 1418–22.

29. Julian TM. The efficacy or Marlex mesh in the repair of severe, recurrent vaginal prolapse of the anterior midvaginal wall. Am J Obstet Gynecol 1996; 175:1472–5.

30. Debodinance P, Berrocal J, Clave H, et al. (Changing attitudes on the surgical treatment of urogenital prolapse: birth of the tension-free vaginal mesh) (Article in French). J Gynecol Obstet Biol Reprod (Paris) 2004; 33(7):577–88.

31. Stanton SL, Hilton P, Norton C, Cardozo L. Clinical and urodynamic effects of anterior colporrhaphy and vaginal hysterectomy for prolapse with and without incontinence. Br J Obstet Gynaecol 1982; 89(6):459–63.

32. Macer GA. Transabdominal repair of cystocele, a 20 year experience, compared with the traditional vaginal approach. Am J Obstet Gynecol 1978; 131(2):203–7.

33. Walter S, Olesen KP, Hald T, Jensen HK, Pedersen PH. Urodynamic evaluation after vaginal repair and colposuspension. Br J Urol 1982; 54(4):377–80.

34. Gardy M, Kozminski M, DeLancey J, Elkins T, McGuire EJ. Stress incontinence and cystoceles. J Urol 1991; 145(6):1211–3.

35. Shull BL, Baden WF. A six-year experience with paravaginal defect repair for urinary stress incontinence. Am J Obstet Gynecol 1989; 160(6):1432–9 (Discussion 1439—40).

36. Shull BL, Benn SJ, Kuehl TJ. Surgical management of prolapse of the anterior vaginal segment: an analysis of support defects, operative morbidity, and anatomic outcome. Am J Obstet Gynecol 1994; 171(6):1429–36 (Discussion 1436—9).

37. Sand PK, Koduri S, Lobel RW, et al. Prospective randomized trial of polyglactin 910 mesh to prevent recurrence of cystoceles and rectoceles. Am J Obstet Gynecol 2001; 184(7):1357–62 (Discussion 1362—4).

38. Weber AM, Walters MD, Piedmonte MR, Ballard LA. Anterior colporrhaphy: a randomized trial of three surgical techniques. Am J Obstet Gynecol 2001; 185 (6):1299–304 (Discussion 1304—6).

39. Nicita G. A new operation for genitourinary prolapse. J Urol 1998; 160:741–5.

40. Flood CG, Drutz HP, Waja L. Anterior colporraphy reinforced with Marlex mesh for the treatment of cystoceles. Int Urogynecol J 1998; 9:200–4.

41. Mage P. Interposition of a synthetic mesh by vaginal approach in the cure of genital prolapse. J Gynecol Obstet Biol Reprod (Paris) 1999; 28(8):825–9.

42. Migliari R, De Angelis M, Madeddu G, Verdacchi T. Tension-free vaginal mesh repair for anterior vaginal wall prolapse. Eur Urol 2000; 38:151–5.

43. Hardiman P, Oyawoye S, Browning J. Cystocele repair using polypropylene mesh. Br J Obstet Gynecol 2000; 107:825–6.

44. Eglin G, Ska JM, Serres X. Transobturator subvesical mesh. Tolerance and short-term results of a 103 case continuous series]. Gynecol Obstet Fertil 2003; 31(1):14–9 (Article in French).
45. Sergent F, Marpeau L. Prosthetic restoration of the pelvic diaphragm in genital urinary prolapse surgery trans-obturator and infracoccygeal hammock technique. J Obstet Gynecol Biol Reprod (Paris) 2003; 32(2):120–6.
46. Adhoute F, Soyeur L, Pariente JL, Le Guillou M, Ferriere JM. Use of transvaginal polypropylene mesh (Gynemesh) for the treatment of pelvic floor disorders in women. Prospective study in 52 patients. Prog Urol 2004; 14(2): 192–6.
47. Shah DK, Paul EM, Rastinehad AR, Eisenberg ER, Baldani GH. Short-term outcome analysis of total pelvis reconstruction with mesh: the vaginal approach. J Urol 2004; 171(1):261–3.
48. Dwyer PL, O'Reilly BA. Transvaginal repair of anterior and posterior compartment prolapse with Atrium polypropylene mesh. Br J Obstet Gynaecol 2004; 111:831–6.
49. Milani R, Salvatore S, Soligo M, Pifarotti P, Meschia M, Cortese M. Functional and anatomical outcome of anterior and posterior vaginal prolapse repair with prolene mesh. Br J Obstet Gynaecol 2004; 111:1–5.
50. de Tayrac R, Gervaise A, Chauveaud A, Fernandez H. Tension-free polypropylene mesh for vaginal repair of anterior vaginal wall prolapse. J Reprod Med 2005; 50(2):75–80.
51. Nygaard IE, McCreery R, Brubaker L, et al. Abdominal sacrocolpopexy: a comprehensive review. Obstet Gynecol 2004; 104(4):805–23.
52. Cruikshank SH. Sacrospinous fixation-should this be performed at the time of vaginal hysterectomy? Am J Obstet Gynecol 1991; 164(4):1072–6.
53. Karram M, Goldwasser S, Kleeman S, Steele A, Vassallo B, Walsh P. High uterosacral vaginal vault suspension with fascial reconstruction for vaginal repair of enterocele and vaginal vault prolapse. Am J Obstet Gynecol 2001; 185 (6):1339–42 (Discussion 1342—3).
54. Lefranc JP, Atallah D, Camatte S, Blondon J. Longterm followup of posthysterectomy vaginal vault prolapse abdominal repair: a report of 85 cases. J Am Coll Surg 2002; 195(3):352–8.
55. Nezhat CH, Nezhat F, Nezhat C. Laparoscopic sacral colpopexy for vaginal vault prolapse. Obstet Gynecol 1994; 84(5):885–8.
56. Cosson M, Rajabally R, Bogaert E, Querleu D, Crepin G. Laparoscopic sacrocolpopexy, hysterectomy, and burch colposuspension: feasibility and short-term complications of 77 procedures. JSLS 2002; 6(2):115–19.
57. Randall CL, Nichols DH. Surgical treatment of vaginal inversion. Obstet Gynecol. 1971; 38(3):327–32.
58. Sze EH, Karram MM. Transvaginal repair of vault prolapse: a review. Obstet Gynecol. 1997; 89(3):466–75.
59. Ho YH, Ang M, Nyam D, Tan M, Seow-Choen F. Transanal approach to rectocele repair may compromise anal sphincter pressures. Dis Colon Rectum 1998; 41(3):354–8.
60. Kahn MA, Stanton SL. Posterior colporrhaphy: its effects on bowel and sexual function. Br J Obstet Gynaecol 1997; 104(1):82–6.

61. Cundiff GW, Weidner AC, Visco AG, Addison WA, Bump RC. An anatomic and functional assessment of the discrete defect rectocele repair. Am J Obstet Gynecol 1998; 179(6 Pt 1):1451–6 (Discussion 1456—7).
62. Porter WE, Steele A, Walsh P, Kohli N, Karram MM. The anatomic and functional outcomes of defect-specific rectocele repairs. Am J Obstet Gynecol 1999; 181(6):1353–8 (Discussion 1358—9).
63. Watson SJ, Loder PB, Halligan S, Bartram CI, Kamm MA, Phillips RK. Transperineal repair of symptomatic rectocele with Marlex mesh: a clinical, physiological and radiologic assessment of treatment. J Am Coll Surg 1996; 183 (3):257–61.
64. Sullivan ES, Longaker CJ, Lee PY. Total pelvic mesh repair: a ten-year experience. Dis Colon Rectum 2001; 44(6):857–63.
65. Von Theobald P, Labbe E. Three-way prosthetic repair of the pelvic floor. J Gynecol Obstet Biol Reprod (Paris) 2003; 32(6):562–70.
66. Maher CF, Qatawneh AM, Dwyer PL, Carey MP, Cornish A, Schluter PJ. Abdominal sacral colpopexy or vaginal sacrospinous colpopexy for vaginal vault prolapse: a prospective randomized study. Am J Obstet Gynecol 2004; 190(1):20–6.
67. Roovers JP, van der Vaart CH, van der Bom JG, van Leeuwen JH, Scholten PC, Heintz AP. A randomised controlled trial comparing abdominal and vaginal prolapse surgery: effects on urogenital function. BJOG 2004; 111(1): 50–6.
68. Meschia M, Pifarotti P, Spennacchio M, Buonaguidi A, Gattei U, Somigliana E. A randomized comparison of tension-free vaginal tape and endopelvic fascia plication in women with genital prolapse and occult urinary stress incontinence. Am J Obstet Gynecol 2004; 190(3):609–13.
69. de Tayrac R, Gervaise A, Chauveaud-Lambling A, Fernandez H. Combined genital prolapse repair reinforced with a polypropylene mesh and tension-free vaginal tape in women with genital prolapse and urinary stress incontinence: a retrospective case-control study with short-term follow-up. Acta Obstet Gynecol Scand 2004; 83(10):950–4.
70. Rogers RG, Kammerer-Doak D, Darrow A, Murray K, Olsen A, Barber M, Qualls C. Sexual function after surgery for urinary stress incontinence and/or pelvic organ prolapse: A multicenter prospective study. Am J Obstet Gynecol 2004; 191:206–10.

8

Paraurethral Injections and Other Options

Pieter J. Verleyen

Department of Urology, AZ Groeninge Hospital, Kortrijk, Belgium

INTRODUCTION

Bulking agents are injected paraurethrally to support the intrinsic sphincter function. Polytetrafluoroethylene (PTFE), commonly known as Teflon®, is the first popular agent, which migrates to lungs and brain and is potentially carcinogenic. Collagen has a rather short effect and is allergenic. Injection of autologous fat can lead to fat embolism. Macroplastique® is a well tolerated, safe, and stable silicone elastomer with good bulking capacity. Deflux® is a dextranomer-hyaluronic acid copolymer with a superior biocompatibility. It is safe, easy to use and approved for children. In the future, injection of stem cells may allow the restoration of a damaged sphincter in humans.

Paraurethral injections are preferentially performed by transurethral (cystoscopic) access. The bulking agent is implanted submucosally in the area of the bladder neck. It augments the urethral mucosa and thus causes a functional lengthening of the urethra. It improves mucosal coaptation and intrinsic sphincter function, gives a better pressure transmission to the proximal urethra and increases urethral closing pressure. As a result, the bladder neck remains closed during stress. New devices allow a three- or four-point injection at a constant position, angle and depth.

Most studies about paraurethral injections are of poor methodological quality. 70% improve postoperatively, with only 30% of patients remaining dry after two years. Side effects are usually mild. Temporarily urinary retention occurs in about 10% of patients.

MATERIAL: BULKING AGENT

Bulking agents are substances that can be injected submucosally and act as a permanent implant. They can be used to treat urinary stress incontinence or vesico-ureteral reflux. The ideal implant should be cost-effective, non-degradable, biologically inert, nontoxic, nonimmunogenic and non-carcinogenic. The agent should be easy to use, keep the original volume and bind to local tissues with minimal inflammation. It may not migrate to other organs and have no influence on later surgery. In order not to migrate, the particle size should exceed 80 µm. The optimal agent probably does not exist yet. Durability is a primary concern with this technique.

In a first report in 1938, a sclerosing solution (sodium morrhuate) was used to inject into the anterior vaginal wall to obtain scarring of the juxta urethral tissue (1). In 1955, Quackels described paraffin injection to treat incontinence (2) and Sachse in 1963 used a slerosing agent Dondren to inject in the urethra (3). These agents all cause local tissue damage and may result in pulmonary emboli and infarction.

Only in the seventies did the technique become popular after reports on PTFE injections by Berg (4) and Politano (5). The injection of Teflon is difficult due to its high viscosity (6). It can lead to scarring and fibrosis and can cause a para-urethral abscess (7). Moreover, migration to lymph nodes, lung, kidney, brain and spleen (6) has been described, with granulomatous inflammations. It may also have a carcinogenic potential (8).

In 1989, glutaraldehyde cross-linked collagen (Contigen®) (9) and autologous fat (10) were introduced as bulking agents. In Contigen®, North American bovine collagen is cross-linked with Glutaraldehyde. It is expensive and rapidly absorbed, repeated injections are often necessary. Because of possible allergy (in 4% of cases), pre-injection skin testing is necessary (11). But this does not exclude late-onsetallergy (with arthralgia, skin reaction, flu-like symptoms). Sterile abscess formation and osteitis pubis were also described. Infection with BSE is a theoretical possibility (12). Autologous fat is rapidly absorbed and repeated injections are necessary. Harvesting of the tissue is painful. One death due to fat embolism was reported and the results were disappointing (13).

In the nineties, other substances were introduced: carbon coated zirconium beads (Durasphere®), polydimethylsiloxane (Macroplastique®), and dextran-hyaluronic acid (Deflux®). Durasphere® can migrate to the lymph nodes and urethral mucosa. The long-term results are not better than for collagen and repeated injections are necessary, but there is no risk of allergy (14).

Macroplastique® is polydimethylsiloxane (a silicone elastomer) suspended in a bio-excretable carrier gel (povidone hydrogel). The gel is absorbed by the reticulo-endothelial system and excreted unchanged in the urine. It is well tolerated by the immune system; it is nontoxic, noncarcinogenic, and nonteratogenic. No migration has been observed (particle size: 120–264 μm). Because of its high viscosity, the injection is more difficult to perform. The irregularly shaped and textured surface of the particles encourages agglomeration and host collagen deposition. It organizes in firm nodules after 6 weeks to 9 months and gets infiltrated by collagen and surrounded by a fibrous sheath. No biodegradation or migration has been found. Because of the good bulking properties, only a small amount of substance is required. Solid polydimethylsiloxane in breast implants can lead to late-onset connective tissue disorders, but this was never found with silicone gel (15).

Deflux® is a co-polymer of dextranomer (cross-linked dextran) and nonanimal stabilized hyaluronic acid, with a superior biocompatibility. Dextran has been used for plasma-expanders and wound dressings. Rare cases of anaphylaxis have been reported with dextran, not with dextranomer. Hyaluronic acid is a universal component of the extra cellular space in all tissues and all species and is used in eye surgery, esthetic treatments and joint injections. It will be replaced by connective tissue. Deflux® does not migrate (particles 80–250 μm), is nonimmunogenic, nontoxic, noncarcinogenic, and nonteratogenic and shows no granuloma formation (17). It cannot be infected by prions, viruses or proteins. It is the only Food and Drug Administration–approved agent for endoscopic treatment of vesicoureteric reflux in children. It remains stable more than 3 years in the urinary system. Fibroblast activity and collagen ingrowth is stimulated by hyaluronic acid. Because of its low viscosity, it is easy to inject. There is a 20% volume-reduction after 1 year. It is probably somewhat less stable than Macroplastique® on the long term.

In the future, injection of stem cells may be an option to treat sphincter incompetence. Tissue engineering in rats has shown some positive results: Autologous or allogenic muscle derived stem cells injected in the sphincter can improve the leak point pressure, form new anatomic motor units and restore deficient sphincter function (17,18).

TECHNIQUE

The injection is preferentially performed via transurethral access. The transvaginal or transperineal approach, even ultrasound-guided, is less successful (19). It can be performed under local anesthesia (transurethral injection of a lidocaine gel) in an outpatient-setting. The special injection needle is inserted through the Albarran cystoscope. Injection of the substance is performed under direct cystoscopic vision between the bladder neck and mid-urethral level. A first and second injection are performed at the 3 and 9 o'clock position, a third at the 6 o'clock position somewhat more distal and deeper than the other implantations. The product is injected until good coalescence of the mucosa is reached. The needle should, after each injection, be left in place for 30 s to avoid leakage of the product. Tunnelling of the needle about 5 mm submucosally before injection limits loss of product and stimulates ingrowth. The bladder should be emptied with a very small calibre of transurethral catheter, in and out to avoid compression of the submucosal bulking agent.

More recently, newer implantation techniques became available: the three-point injection technique with the Macroplastique Implantation Device™ (MID) or the four-point technique with the Zuidex Implacer™ (Deflux®). These devices allow an implantation with three or four needles at a constant depth, angle and position and this in the same circumferential plane. This results in an easier and more accurate positioning of the bulking agent. Experience is still limited, but the initial results seem promising (20,21) (Fig. 1).

INDICATIONS

This technique is valuable for women with stress incontinence due to intrinsic sphincter incontinence. It can also be offered to women whose incontinence is associated with bladder neck mobility and where a suspension or a sling procedure had insufficient results. It is a good option, especially in elderly women with a high operative risk, in patients who refuse open surgery, or after multiple pelvic surgery or radiotherapy. In women with stress incontinence who whish to become pregnant, a sling operation can cause problems for normal delivery. These patients can also benefit from paraurethral injections (15,22). The technique can be offered to children with a structural incontinence (e.g., after correction of bladder exstrophy) (23) or to girls with therapy-resistant daytime-incontinence and an insufficient bladder neck (typically with leakage in the afternoon or giggle-incontinence) (24). Women with overactive bladder contractions, important bladder neck mobility and gross pelvic organ prolapse are no good candidates for this procedure. In case of doubt, a video-urodynamic investigation is advised.

RESULTS

It is difficult to interpret the results of incontinence procedures because of the poor methodological quality of most studies. Almost no prospective randomized comparisons between different techniques or bulking agents exist. Most studies include patients with a variety of indications and often women with previous incontinence or prolapse surgery. The number of injections and volume injected differ between different studies and the follow-up period is usually short (15,25). In most studies, the effect decreases over time.

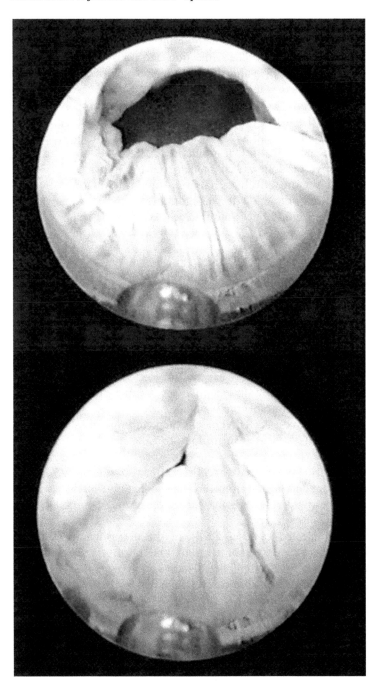

Figure 1 Cystoscopic view during a paraurethral injection showing the submucosal needle and the mucosal bulging effect (*bottom*) after the injection.

With Macroplastique®, one can expect an improvement rate of about 70% after 6 months and 50% after 2 years with about 45% of dry patients after 6 months and 30% after 2 years. The reinjection rate after 6 months is about 33% (15). The results are worse and there is a higher rate of complications when a paraurethral access is used (19,25).

Using the Zuidex™, the first reports show improvement in 77% after one year (21). With the MID, the 2 year improvement rate is about 70% (20). Both of these techniques show a significant quality of life improvement as assessed by the King's Health Questionnaire (20,22).

In a prospective randomized controlled trial by Maher et al. (26), a pubovaginal sling is more effective than transurethral Macroplastique®: 69% versus 21% are continent after 62 months. Macroplastique® has a significantly lower morbidity but is more expensive than the sling.

COMPLICATIONS

The technique-related complications are mild and transient: Dysuria, frequency, de novo instability, hematuria, pain and infection occur in less than 10% of the subjects. Urinary retention requiring timely intermittent catheterization can occur in about 10%.

BOTULINUM TOXIN INTRADETRUSOR INJECTION

Intradetrusor injection of botulinum toxin is an increasingly popular treatment for patients with an overactive bladder syndrome. Intramuscular injection of Botulinum toxin A (BTA) blocks the neuromuscular junction at the site of injection. BTA is used in urology to treat neurogenic detrusor overactivity, chronic urinary retention, detrusor-sphincter dyssynergia, nonneurogenic detrusor overactivity and pelvic floor spasticity (1–5). Only the application in patients with a nonneurogenic overactive bladder will be discussed here. These patients present with urgency and eventually urge incontinence.

The toxin is injected cystoscopically in the detrusor-muscle. BTA injection reduces the overactive contractions and results in a significant higher bladder capacity and compliance. There are no general side effects. Urinary retention can occur in rare cases. The effect of the treatment lasts about 9 months.

MATERIAL: BOTULINUM TOXIN

Botulinum toxin is the neurotoxin from the Clostridium botulinum bacterium that causes the food related poisoning called botulism. It is a selective blocker of acetylcholine release by binding to the presynaptic nerve-endings. In a striated muscle, the neuromuscular junction is then blocked until new pre-synaptic nerve sprouts occur. This process takes approximately 2 to 4 months at the mammalian neuromuscular junction, but up to 1 year in autonomic neurones (6). In the detrusor muscle, this process is not yet fully understood and the recuperation process may be different (7). Two botulinum toxin antigenic subtypes are in clinical use: type A and B. Type A is the most popular product, because it is more potent and has a longer duration of action. Two commercially available BTA products are used in urology: Botox® (Allergan) and Dysport® (Ipsen). It is generally considered that 1 U of Botox® is equivalent to 3 to 4 U of Dysport® (8).

TECHNIQUE

The toxin is diluted in saline and injected cystoscopically at 15 to 30 sites in the detrusor, avoiding the trigone and ureteral orifices (to prevent vesico–ureteral reflux). The procedure is performed under general or loco regional anesthesia in a day-case setting. Mostly, a dose of 200 to 300 U of Botox (or the equivalent dose of Dysport) is injected. Postoperatively, the patients should be followed with special attention to the possible development of post void residual urine. Patients have a good symptom relief after 2 weeks.

INDICATIONS

BTA is used in neurogenic and nonneurogenic voiding dysfunctions. Patients with an overactive bladder syndrome are good candidates for BTA treatment if anticholinergics are not effective enough or cause too many side effects. These patients are sometimes treated without a uro-dynamic confirmation of the presumed diagnosis, detrusor overactivity. The patients present with urgency and eventually urge incontinence, usually with frequency and nocturia (4). In children with a therapy-resistant detrusor overactivity, BTA showed to be safe and effective. It reduces the overactive contractions (associated with urgency) and increases the bladder capacity (3).

RESULTS

All the studies show an impressive increase in functional bladder capacity and a reduction in overactive bladder contractions. BTA reduces the urgency symptoms and the number of incontinence episodes (1,4). There is an important variability in the results in terms of the efficacy and longevity of the treatment. One of the reasons is that both the optimum dose of BTA and the number of injection sites is not known. Studies assessing the impact on quality of life are also lacking (4). The effect of the treatment seems to last for about 9 months (1,3,4). There is also no decline in the benefit of repeat administrations and there are no definitive ultra structural changes in the detrusor muscle (7,9).

COMPLICATIONS

Side effects are very rare. Injection of BTA results in a less active detrusor and can therefore lead to post void residual urine and even urinary retention. Residual urine can cause urinary tract infections. It is advisable to measure the post void residue after two weeks. In the rare case of urinary retention, intermittent catheterization is necessary.

General contraindications for BTA are myasthenia gravis, intake of aminoglycosides or other drugs that interfere with neuromuscular transmission, breastfeeding and coagulation disorders. The injected dose is about 1/1000 of the lethal dose in an average 70 kg person. Only a fraction of the locally injected dose reaches the systemic circulation. Only two cases of general weakness have been reported. But the authors speculated that the cumulative dose was probably too high in one patient and the product may have diffused through the thin bladder wall in the other patient, allowing more resorption intraabdominally (10).

REFERENCES

1. Murless BC. The injection treatment of stress incontinence. J Obstet Gynaecol Br Emp 1938; 45:67–71.
2. Quackels R. Deux incontinences après adenomectomie guéries par injection de paraffine dans le perinee. Acta Urol Belg 1955; 23:259–62.
3. Sachse S. Treatment of urinary incontinence with sclerosing agent solutions: indication, results, complications. Urol Int 1963; 15:225–44.
4. Berg S. Polytef augmentation urethroplasty correction of surgically incurable incontinence by injection technique. Arch Surg 1973; 107:379–81.
5. Politano AV. Periurethral polytetafluoroethylene injection for urinary incontinence. J Urol 1982; 127:439–42.
6. Mittleman RE, Maracchini JV. Pulmonary Teflon granuloma following periurethral Teflon injection for urinary incontinence. Arch Pathol Lab Med 1983; 107:611–18.
7. Kiilholma PJ, Chancellor MB, Makinen J, et al. Complications of Teflon injection for urinary stress incontinence. Neurourol Urodyn 1993; 12:131–7.
8. Hakky M, Kolbusz R, Reyes CV. Chondrosarcoma of the larynx. Ear Nose Throat J 1989; 68:60–2.
9. Shortliffe LMD, Freiha FS, Kessler R, et al. Treatment of urinary incontinence by periurethral implantation of glutaraldehyde cross-linked collagen. J Urol 1989; 141:538–41.
10. Gonzales de Garibay S, Jimeno C, et al. Endoscopic autotransplantation of fat tissue in the treatment of urinary incontinence in the female. J d'Urol 1989; 95: 363–6.

11. Appell RA. Collagen injection therapy for urinary incontinence. Urol Clin North Am 1994; 21:177–82.
12. Stothers L, Goldenberg SL, Leone EF. Complications of periurethral collagen injection for urinary stress incontinence. J Urol 1998; 159:806–7.
13. Currie L, Drutz HP, Oxorn D. Adipose tissue and lipid drop embolism following periurethral injection of autologous fat: case report and review of the litterature. Int Urogynecol J Pelvic Floor Dysfunct 1997; 8:923–6.
14. Pannek J, Brands FH, Senge T. Particle migration after transurethral injection of carbon coated beads for urinary stress incontinence. J Urol 2001; 166(4): 1350–3.
15. ter Meulen PH, Berghmans LC, van Kerrebroeck PE. Systematic review: efficacy of silicone microimplants (Macroplastique) therapy for urinary stress incontinence in adult women. Eur Urol 2003; 44(5):573–82.
16. Stenberg A, Lackgren G. A new bioimplant for the endoscopic treatment of vesicoureteral reflux: experimental and short-term clinical results. J Urol 1995; 154(2):800–3.
17. Cannon TW, Lee JY, Somogyi G, et al. Improved sphincter contractility after allogenic muscle-derived progenitor cell injection into the denervated rat urethra. Urology 2003; 62(5):958–63.
18. Yiou R, Yoo JJ, Atala A. Restoration of functional motor units in a rat model of sphincter injury by muscle precursor cell autografts. Transplantation 2003; 76(7):1053–60.
19. Gottfried HW, Maier S, Gschwend J, et al. Minimally invasive treatment of urinary stress incontinence by collagen administration. Comparison between endosonography controlled and transurethral submucous collagen injection. Urologe A 1996; 35(1):6–10.
20. Tamanini JT, D'Ancona CA, Netto NR Jr. Treatment of intrinsic sphincter deficiency using the Macroplastique Implantation System: two-year follow-up. J Endourol 2004; 18(9):906–11.
21. Chapple CR, Haab F, Cervigni M, et al. An open, multicentre study of NASHA/Dx Gel (Zuidex™) for the treatment of urinary stress incontinence. Eur Urol 2005, Jun 17 (E-pub ahead of print).
22. van Kerrebroeck P, ter Meulen F, Farrelly E, et al. Treatment of urinary stress incontinence: recent developments in the role of urethral injection. Urol Res 2003; 30(6):356–62.
23. Lottmann HB, Margaryan M, Bernuy M, et al. The effect of endoscopic injections of dextranomer based implants on continence and bladder capacity: a prospective study of 31 patients. J Urol 2002; 168(4):1863–7.
24. Läckgren G, Lottmann H, Hensle T, et al. Endoscopic treatment of vesicoureteral reflux and urinary incontinence in children. AUA Update Series 2003; 22:294–299.
25. Pickard R, Reaper J, Wyness L, et al. Periurethral injection therapy for urinary incontinence in women. Cochrane Database Syst Rev. 2003; (2):CD003881.
26. Maher CF, O'Reilly BA, Dwyer PL, et al. Pubovaginal sling versus transurethral Macroplastique for urinary stress incontinence and intrinsic sphincter deficiency: a prospective randomized controlled trial. BJOG 2005; 112(6):797–801.

27. Leippold T, Reitz A, Schurch B. Botulinum toxin as a new therapy option for voiding disorders: current state of the art. Eur Urol 2003; 44(2):165–74.
28. Schulte-Baukloh H, Michael T, Schobert J,, et al. Efficacy of botulinum-a toxin in children with detrusor hyperreflexia due to myelomeningocele: preliminary results. Urology 2002; 59(3):325–7.
29. Verleyen P, Hoebeke P, Raes A, et al. The use of Botulinum Toxin A in children with a non-neurogenic overactive bladder: a pilot study. BJUI 2004; 93(Suppl. 2):69.
30. Sahai A, Khan M, Fowler CJ, et al. Botulinum toxin for the treatment of lower urinary tract symptoms: a review. Neurourol Urodyn 2005; 24(1):2–12.
31. Schurch B, de Seze M, Denys P, et al. Botox Detrusor Hyperreflexia Study Team. Botulinum toxin type a is a safe and effective treatment for neurogenic urinary incontinence: results of a single treatment, randomized, placebo controlled 6-month study. J Urol 2005; 174(1):196–200.
32. Naumann M, Jost WH, Toyka KV. Botulinum toxin in the treatment of neurological disorders of the autonomic nervous system. Arch Neurol 1999; 56(8):914–16.
33. Haferkamp A, Schurch B, Reitz A, et al. Lack of ultrastructural detrusor changes following endoscopic injection of botulinum toxin type a in overactive neurogenic bladder. Eur Urol 2004; 46(6):784–91.
34. Odergren T, Hjaltason H, Kaakkola S, et al. A double blind, randomised, parallel group study to investigate the dose equivalence of Dysport and Botox in the treatment of cervical dystonia. J Neurol Neurosurg Psychiatry 1998; 64(1):6–12.
35. Gross J, Kramer G, Schurch B, et al. Repeated injections of Botulinum-A toxin in patients with neurogenic lower urinary tract dysfunction do not cause increased drug tolerance. Neurourol Urodyn 2002; 21(4):386–7.
36. Wyndaele JJ, Van Dromme SA. Muscular weakness as side effect of botulinum toxin injection for neurogenic detrusor overactivity. Spinal Cord 2002; 40(11): 599–600.

9

Computer-Based Electronic Artificial Sphincters

Kathleen D'Hauwers

University Medical Center, St. Radboud, Nijmegen, The Netherlands

HISTORY

One of the surgical treatments for urinary stress incontinence is simulating the function of the native sphincter by an artificial genito-urinary sphincter (AGUS) (1). The first AGUS was designed in 1947 by Foley and consisted of an occlusive periurethral cuff. Brantley Scott did the first implant in a human in 1972 in a 36-year-old woman with spina bifida and myelomeningocele. This model 721 was made of silicone rubber and consisted of four components: a reservoir, an inflatable occlusive cuff, an inflate bulb (right side), and a deflate bulb (left side). The pressure was regulated by a mechanical V4 valve, which allowed a maximal pressure of 80 to 90 cm H_2O in the inflatable cuff. The disadvantages of the AS 721, leading to a high rate of mechanical failure, included the two-pump-mechanism, the V4 valve for pressure regulation, lack of automatic cuff closure and the technically difficult operation.

The next model, AGUS 761 incorporated a pressure-regulating balloon between valve and cuff. Later, model 742 (1974) had the first automatic cuff closure prosthesis consisting of a single pump, a cuff and a balloon pressure reservoir which replaced the V4 valve. The combination of active pressure in the regulating balloon and the delay fill resistor made the automatic but slow return of fluid to the cuff possible.

Models AS 791-792 (1979: 791-bulbous urethral placement/792-bladder neck placement) consisted of an inflatable cuff, a pressure-regulating balloon reservoir, a pump and a control assembly. In model 791, a dip-coated all-silicone rubber cuff replaced the Dacron-reinforced cuff, and the control assembly combined the valves and resistor within a stainless steel case. This resulted in fewer connections and in an easier surgical procedure. However, since the device could not be deactivated except during the times the patient would void, the constant pressure on the urethra led to relatively high rates of cuff erosion. This led to the concept of "delayed activation" by Furlow (2) in 1999. Placing the components but leaving the ends of the tubing plugged, leaving the pump and reservoir full of fluid and the cuff empty, performed deactivation. Six to twelve weeks later, through a small inguinal incision, the three components were connected to the cylindrical valve mechanisms, activating the device.

The AS 800 (1983), the most commonly used AGUS today, resembles model 791 but the control assembly incorporates a deactivation button/valve and is, with the refill resistor, joined with the deflation pump as one component. The device can be activated without a second surgical procedure. The material, however, still causes problems. Placed and inflated around the urethra, the cuff assumes a polygonal shape. Deflated silicone cuffs develop folds that remain to some extent during inflation. Furthermore, while the cuffs are deflated, the silicone shell comes in contact with the Dacron backing. Molecules tend to migrate and cause thinning over time and with repeated use. These characteristics, respectively called "silicone memory" and "secondary creep phenomenon," weaken the silicone, leading to fracture and to subsequent leakage.

In 1983 a lubricant surface (fluorosilicone) was introduced onto the cuff to diminish the potential weakening of the silicone at the cuff folds. Additionally, in 1988 the "narrow-back cuff principle" was introduced. The diameter of the outer polypropylene backing of the cuff was decreased from 2 to 1.5 cm; the inner cuff shell was maintained at a width of 2 cm. This allows expansion of the inner cuff along a greater urethral length, improving the transmission of cuff pressure to the underlying tissue and decreasing the incidence of secondary tissue pressure atrophy and cuff erosion.

Finally, the current model 800 consists of (*i*) control assembly/pump combining two valves, one resistor, and a deactivation button; (*ii*) surface-treated urethral cuff made of silicone elastomers (12 sizes ranging from 4.0 to 11 cm long) that consists of an outer monofilament of knitted polypropylene (Dacron) backing and an inner silicone leaflet that is in contact with the urethra (2.0 cm wide when deflated); (*iii*) kink-resistant and color-coded tubing (the control pump tubing that connects to the cuff tubing has clear nylon filament inside and the control pump tubing that connects to the balloon tubing has black nylon filament inside); and (*iv*) pressure-controlling balloon reservoir that comes in various pressure ranges (41 to 50, 51 to 60, 61 to 70, 71 to 80, and 81 to 90 cm H_2O).

Many different materials (3), including solid silicone elastomers, are associated with malignant tumor formation in laboratory animals, but only with implants of relatively large size. No such effect has been described in humans. Extensive testing of all materials of the AMS 800 (American Medical Systems, Inc., Minnetonka, Minnesota, U.S.A.) indicated no toxicological response. Some of the materials caused only minor irritation when implanted in animals. Silicone elastomer shedding and migrating to regional lymph nodes has been reported in the literature on penile implants.

MECHANISM

The prosthesis consists of three components (4): an occlusive cuff implanted around the bladder neck (♀,♀) or the bulbous urethra (♀), a pressure-regulating balloon implanted in the prevesical space and a control pump implanted in the labia major or the hemiscrotum (Fig. 1). All components are interconnected with color-coded, kink-resistant tubing. The cuff of the AGUS occludes the urethra preventing urine from passing (Fig. 2). When the patient wants to void, he squeezes and releases the control pump several times. This transfers the fluid from the cuff to the pressure-regulating balloon (Fig. 3). The cuff flattens allowing the urine to flow from the

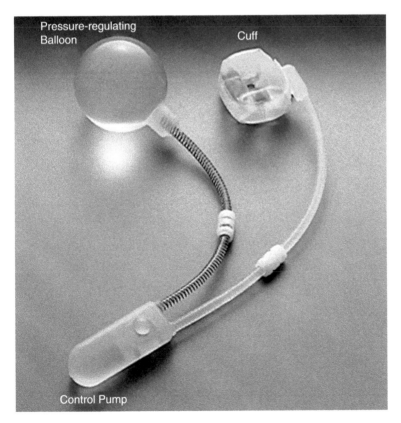

Figure 1 The AMS 800. Implantable fluid-filled solid silicone elastomer with three components: occlusive cuff, pressure regulating balloon, control pump, color-coded tubing. *Source*: American Medical Systems, Inc.

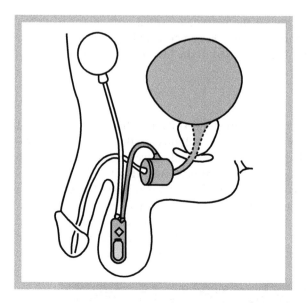

Figure 2 The cuff of the AGUS occludes the urethra, preventing urine from passing. *Source*: American Medical Systems, Inc.

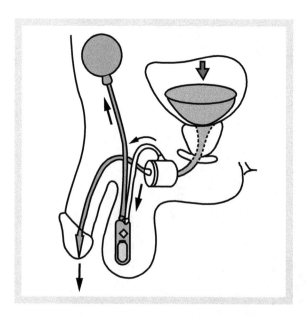

Figure 3 Squeezing and releasing the control pump several times transfers the fluid from the cuff to the pressure-regulating balloon. The cuff flattens allowing the urine to flow from the bladder through the urethra. *Source*: American Medical Systems, Inc.

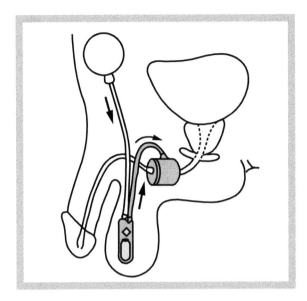

Figure 4 Within several minutes, the pressure-regulating balloon automatically returns the fluid to the cuff to occlude the urethra. *Source*: American Medical Systems, Inc.

bladder through the urethra. Within several minutes, the pressure-regulating balloon automatically returns the fluid to the cuff to occlude the urethra (Fig. 4). Filling solutions include Hypaque (50 mL radiopaque contrast medium with 60 mL sterile water), Cysto-Conray II (60/15 mL), and Urovist Cysto (50/50 mL) (1). In patients who have had an adverse reaction to radio-opaque solutions, isotonic saline should be used.

INDICATION AND PATIENT SELECTION

Indication is urinary stress incontinence due to reduced outlet resistance. The AGUS can be implanted in patients with neurological and non-neurological related incontinence, in adults and in children (Table 1).

Table 1 Indications for Use of AGUS

Neurological	Non-neurological
Spinal cord injury	Post-surgery (prostatectomy, hysterectomy, cystectomy)
Meningomyelocele	Lower urinary tract reconstruction (extrophia/epispadia)
Sacral agenesia	Intrinsic sphincter failure
Spina bifida	Radiotherapy
Severe pelvic trauma	Post non–genito-urinary surgery

Preoperative requirements to the placement of the device are: *i*) urinary incontinence (1,4) should be present for at least 6 months and resistant to conservative therapies, and *ii*) the following preoperative urological conditions are met: *a*) the ability to empty a bladder capacity of at least 200 cc with a urine flow greater than 10 mL/s. The purpose of the implantation is to mimic a normal micturition pattern. Since the urethra will be occluded by the AGUS, the bladder has to be compliant enough to storage a significant volume of urine. When the bladder is fibrotic or overactive, there is no gain in comfort for the patient when he has to handle the pump every 30 minutes. A minimum of detrusor contraction helps to empty the bladder in one cycle. Sometimes the patient has to perform the cycle a few times before the bladder is completely empty. *b*) The urine should be sterile. *c*) Lower abdominal and pelvic integument should be healthy. *d*) The patient should have good manual dexterity and mental faculties to be able to use the device correctly. *e*) He or she should be motivated and have realistic postoperative expectations. The patients must be made aware that the AGUS is not considered to be a lifetime implant; risks for explantation are infection of the device, malfunctioning, and pain.

Some patients continue to have a degree of incontinence after the procedure and become dissatisfied by the presence of a prosthetic device in their body.

Therefore, proper patient selection is of utmost importance. This requires a thorough history (patients with a history of personality disorders should be excluded), a physical examination, urinalysis, urine gram stain and culture, cystoscopy, urodynamic (leak point pressure) and radiographic studies, free flow and postvoid residual urine check, and appropriate consultations as necessary. Tissue fibrosis or previous surgery in the area of implant may preclude application of the device. Bladder neck contractures or urethral strictures can be treated synchronously with the placement of the AGUS (5). Absolute contraindications are an irreversibly obstructed lower urinary tract and irresolvable detrusor overactivity. Problems that affect manual dexterity (as well mental conditions such as dementia as physical conditions such as multiple sclerosis) or motivation may prevent the patient from properly operating the prosthesis. Acute urinary tract infection can interfere with proper functioning of the device and may lead to erosion of the urethra in the cuff area. Poor bladder compliance or a small fibrotic bladder may require an additional intervention such as an augmentation cystoplasty. Of course patients should be fit enough to undergo anaesthesia (Table 2).

PROCEDURE

In both men and women preoperative antibiotic prophylaxis is used. The operative site (abdomen, external genitalia and perineum) is prepared

Table 2 Patient Selection

Conditions
  Present >6 months, resistant to conservative therapy
  Good hand dexterity
  Good mental faculties, motivated, realistic
  Bladder capacity >200 cc
  Qmax >10 mL/s
  Complete bladder emptying must be possible
  Urine: sterile
Contraindications
  Physical/mental conditions
  Irreversibly obstructed lower urinary tract
  Irresolvable detrusor overactivity
  Progressive degenerative disease
Increased risks
  Proven sensitivity to silicone
  Recurrent urinary tract infections
  Diabetes
  Open sores
  Skin infections in the surgical region
  Spinal cord injury
  Scarring (surgery/radiotherapy)

with a 10-min scrub; the patient is draped and catheterised. In women the procedure is performed through a suprapubic incision (dorsal decubitus position) or transvaginally (lithotomy position); in men through a suprapubic incision with a perineal approach (lithotomy position) (3). Recently, the use of a transverse scrotal incision has been described (6). The most important part of the procedure is to locate and dissect the urethra. In women the dissection can be facilitated by a vaginal pack (1). Since all AS 800 cuffs are 2 cm wide, a 2 cm wide plane must be created around the urethra. Before measuring the urethral circumference the transurethral catheter is removed. The cuff is prepared for the implantation by injecting the filling solution into the cuff, aspirating all of the air, and evacuating the fluid again from the cuff. The cuff is placed peri-urethrally. The balloon is prepared by inflating it with approximately 20 cc of solution, aspirating the air, and evacuating the fluid again. The balloon is placed in the prevesical space (Figs. 5 and 6). Both tubings are passed to each other. After flushing the tubing ends, the balloon is filled with 22 cc of filling solution. The cuff tubing and balloon tubing are temporarily connected to allow the cuff to pressurize. After approximately 30s, the tubings are clamped and the connector is removed. The clamps stay in place until all final connections are made.

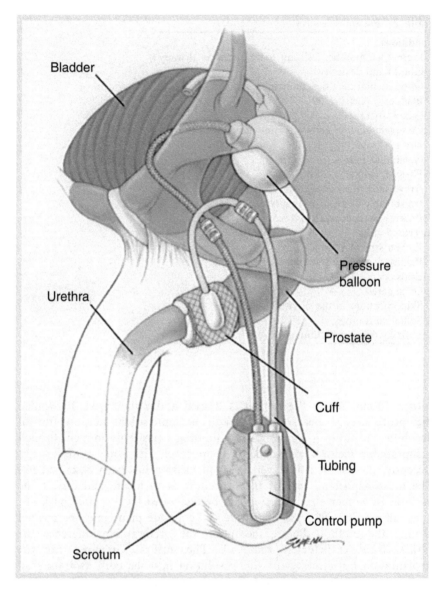

Figure 5   Placement of AGUS, male. *Source*: American Medical Systems, Inc.

From the abdominal incision the right or left hemiscrotum/labium major is dissected for the placement of the pump. The pump should be placed on the same side of the pressure-regulating balloon. After filling the pump with filling solution, it is placed in the scrotum/labium (through the abdominal incision). The pump is placed so that it is easily palpated,

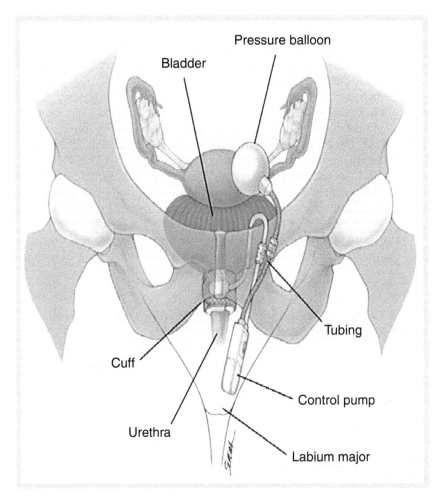

Figure 6   Placement of ANGUS, female. *Source*: American Medical Systems, Inc.

with the deactivation button facing outward. Excess tubing is trimmed and all tubing is connected (tubing with clear nylon filament inside between pump and cuff, tubing with black nylon inside between pump and balloon). The skin can be closed with suture or skin staples. The device should be deactivated for 4 to 6 weeks. To deactivate, the pump is squeezed and released several times to empty the cuff. When the pump has refilled to the point that there is a slight dimple in it, the deactivation button is pushed to lock the cuff open during the healing process. After six weeks the device is activated by giving the pump bulb a firm forceful squeeze.

RESULTS

The most important reason for reduced outlet resistance in men is radical post-prostatectomy status; in women it is intrinsic sphincter deficiency status after failed surgical repair.

Concerning post-prostatectomy incontinence, a prospective, multi-center, nonrandomized clinical study was conducted (3) on 85 patients in whom AMS 800 implants were used. Of these, 26 reported 43 adverse events (Table 3). Of the adverse events, 62.7% were surgery related, 23.3% were device, and 14% were result related. Fourteen patients (16.5%) had 15 revisions up to 24 months following the implant, mostly due to mechanical malfunction ($n = 3$, 3.5%), recurrent incontinence ($n = 2$, 2.4%), erosion ($n = 2$, 2.4%), and infection ($n = 2$, 2.4%). Four of these 14 patients wanted to have their device removed; the other 10 wanted a reimplantation.

The safety end-point was a five-year revision-free rate equivalent to 75%: the probability in this study to remain revision-free during 24 months

Table 3   Results of Prospective Study on AMS 800 ($n = 85$) Post-Prostatectomy Patients: Adverse Events Reported by 26 Patients

	Device	Surgery	Result
Related %	23.3	62.7	14
Impaired device function	7		
Difficult activation	2		
Difficult deactivation	1		
Pain/discomfort		6	
Delayed wound healing		5	
Bladder spasms		2	
Migration		3	
Tissue erosion		2	
Infection		2	
Fistula formation		1	
Hematoma		1	
Swelling		2	
Hydrocele		1	
Tissue Erosion/Infection		1	
Wound Infection		1	
Recurrent incontinence			3
Patient dissatisfaction			1
Positional incontinence			1
Urinary retention			1

Table 4　Physician and Patient Assessment of Post-Implant Incontinence

| | Continence assessment (%) | | | |
| | Physician | | Patient | |
	Dry	Protection	Dry	Protection
1-yr follow-up	63.6	34.1	61.7	36.7
2-yr follow-up	73.3	23.3	65.9	31.7

was 79.5%. Mean device survival rate is 67% at 5 years follow-up. Furthermore, the effect of the prosthesis on the patient's quality of life and the reduction in Incontinence Impact Score from pre-to-post-implant status was evaluated: the pre-implant score was significantly ($p > 0.0001$) higher than the mean scores at all follow-up visits (6, 12, 18, and 24 months). There existed no significant difference between the physician's and the patient's assessment of their incontinence (Table 4). During the postoperative follow-up period no significant difference in health status score was observed; post-implant there was clearly more positive self-esteem (Table 5). Similar results concerning the results, the complications, and the impact on quality of life have been reported (7,8).

　　In women, appropriate work-up and diagnosis for type III urinary stress incontinence is crucial (9). For patients with urethral sphincter deficiency, sling procedures have proved to be the most effective treatment, but they lead to a high rate of urinary retention, especially when there is also detrusor hypotonia. The AGUS is indicated for women with multiple failed anti-incontinence operations, including the suburethral sling procedure. It does not have a role in incontinence treatment secondary to urethral hypermobility. The success rates vary from 68% to 100%. Infections occur in 3% to 7%, erosions in 7% to 29% (9–14). Overall, 37% of the prostheses are removed due to infection or erosion in a 10-year period, with the highest risk in women (56%) and the lowest in men with a bulbar sphincter (23%) (15). This is probably due to the female urethra being thinner than the male

Table 5　Post-Implant Health Status and Self-Esteem

	Health status[a]	Self-esteem[b]
Pre-implant	596	3.5
Post-implant	612	4.1

[a] Health Status Questionnaire: assessment of non-illness–specific parameters: physical functioning, social functioning, energy/fatigue, pain, health perception, and emotional problems.
[b] Rosenberg Self-Esteem Questionnaire: Range from 0 to 6.

urethra and the somewhat more difficult approach of the female bladder neck. Previous surgery or other trauma to the bladder neck is probably an extra risk factor.

In the treatment of patients with neurogenic bladders, the AGUS also has its role. Often (one-third of the cases) the implantation is combined with an augmentation cystoplasty (16). The question is whether the AGUS should be placed at the same time of the augmentation or initially, in a staged manner. Infection ratio when performed simultaneously varies (8–20%) (16–19). When place in a staged manner the highest infection rate is 9.5% (20). With both AGUS and augmentation cystoplasty, clean intermittent self-catheterization is necessary to empty the bladder. A complete overview is presented in Table 6 (7,11,15–19,21–29).

Table 6   Overview

Author (year)	Patients (n)	Infection (%)	Erosion (%)	Mechanical failure (%)	Dry (%)
Patients with Preoperative Radiotherapy					
Martins (1995)	34	NR	8	6	70
Wang (1992)	16	NR	13	13	56
Perez (1992)	11	0	9	NR	36
Gundian (1989)	20	NR	10	NR	83
Marks (1989)	10	NR	20	NR	81
Post-Prostatectomy Patients					
Elliott (1998)	160	2	1	9	79
Litwiller (1996)	65	6	3	NR	44
Singh (1996)	28	10	0	NR	86
Gundian (1989)	117	3	7	16	83
Marks (1989)	16	5	8	NR	81
Type III Incontinence Females					
Webster (1992)	24	0	0	17	92
Appell (1988)	34	0	0	10	100
Diokno (1987)	32	3	0	21	91
Light (1985)	39	3	8	35	92
Patients with Neurogenic Bladder					
Miller (1998)	29	7	0	17	100
Singh (1994)	90	7	8	12	92
Gonzalez (1995)	19	NR	0	NR	84
Strawbridge (1989)	18	5	11	17	100

Abbreviation: NR, not recorded.

COMPLICATIONS

Table 7 provides an overview of possible complications. The most important are discussed below. The outflow resistance created by the cuff is approximately 60 to 70 cm H_2O. This can lead to urethral ischemia, to urethral necrosis and finally to erosion of the device. To overcome this problem a new manufacturing process with several adaptations was developed of which the "narrow backing cuff" (1988) was the most important one in reducing surgical reinterventions. As described above the supportive backing cuff was made narrower than the fluid cuff (reduction from 2 to 1.5 cm), allowing a more even distribution of the occlusive pressure. A retrospective study (30) compared 139 patients with a pre-narrow backing cuff with 184 patients with a narrow backing cuff. Minimum follow-up time was 18 months, there was only one surgeon. The total group consisted of 313 men and 10 women, having 272 sphincters placed at the urethra and 51 at the bladder neck. Forty-two percent of the pre-narrow backing cuff group versus 17% of the narrow backing cuff group required a first reoperation. Mechanical versus non-mechanical failure occurred in 21% vs. 17% with the pre-narrow backing and in 7.6% vs. 9% with the narrow backing cuff (Table 8).

Hypovascularity and fibrosis of the urethra after radiation therapy of the pelvis leads to 10% higher erosion rates (21–25). To lower the rate of radiation-associated complications the cuff should be placed on an endoscopically healthy-appearing urethral segment and a lower pressure balloon reservoir (51–60 cm H_2O) should be used. Primary and nocturnal

Table 7 Post-Operative Complications

Human-related	Device-related
De novo urge	Migration
Retention	Malfunctioning pump, tube kinking
Infection	Leakage
Rejection	
Pain	
Fistula-Diverticulas	
Erosion due to infection:	
Pressure on/damage of the tissue	
Improper cuff sizing	
Improper balloon selection	
Component misplacement:	
Cuff around urethra/bladder neck	
Control pump through scrotum/ labium major	
Balloon into bladder	

Table 8   Reoperation Rates

	Patients (*n*%)		
	Reoperation 1	Reoperation 2	Reoperation 3
Pre–narrow backing cuff	58/139 (42)	18/58 (31)	6/18 (33)
Narrow backing cuff	31/184 (17)	7/31 (23)	1/7 (14)
Total	89/323 (28)	25/89 (28)	7/25 (28)

deactivation is also contributive. There are no radiation-associated risks with previous external beam radiotherapy or brachytherapy (22).

Infection that resists antibiotic therapy results in removal of the prosthesis. Explantation of the device may result in scarring, making a subsequent reimplantation more difficult. The treating physician, based on the patient's medical condition and history, determines the timing of reimplantation. Pain can be experienced when the device is activated and during the period of initial use. When the pain becomes a chronic problem it requires further medical intervention. Mechanical failures, such as all fluid leaks, tube kinking, pump malfunctioning, and connector separations, also lead to surgical intervention. Some individuals choose to deactivate the sphincter at night. The mechanical reliability of the AGUS is not adversely affected by nocturnal deactivation (30). Mechanical failure can occur at any time.

SIMULTANEOUS IMPLANT SURGERY: AGUS—PENILE PROSTHESIS

Implanting both devices simultaneously in patients with urinary stress incontinence and erectile dysfunction is feasible. The AGUS is implanted before the penile prosthesis with the two reservoirs placed in contralateral positions (31). If one implant develops a postoperative infection, only the infected implant has to be removed (32).

Tandem Cuff AGUS

There are reports in literature of a second cuff placement in males secondary to continued incontinence after placement of a standard single-cuff AGUS. Eighty percent of these patients are satisfied after the second implant (33). In men with severe incontinence, initial placement of a dual cuff is an option (34).

AGUS and Pregnancy

The implantation of an AGUS does not cause dyspareunia or compromised fertility (27,35). It is generally accepted to deactivate the AGUS during the 3rd trimester of pregnancy to diminish the excessive pressure on the cuff and bladder neck (36). When this is socially not possible, this should be done at labor and delivery. Broad-spectrum antibiotics should be administered during the perinatal period. The choice of vaginal versus caesarean delivery is the choice of the obstetrician and the patient: both methods are successfully described (36,36). Even with a well functioning sphincter, pregnant women experience the classic voiding problems of pregnancy: urinary frequency and slight incontinence (35).

The Future

Preventing erosion is the challenge when implanting sphincters. The many changes in manufacturing process (since 1972) and especially the design of the narrow backing cuff (since 1987) have led to a drastic reduction in postoperative surgical interventions. In 2002 the fine-tuned sensor controlled artificial sphincter was presented (37). Between cuff and pressure regulating balloon an actuator with a reaction time lower than 10 ms is placed. This microprocessor delivers a continuous peri-urethral pressure that can be increased or decreased according to the needs of the moment (Figs. 7 and 8).

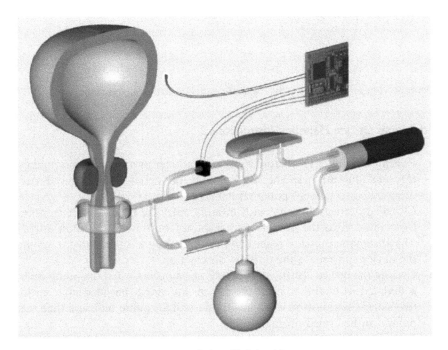

Figure 7 Fine-tuned sensor-controlled artificial sphincter.

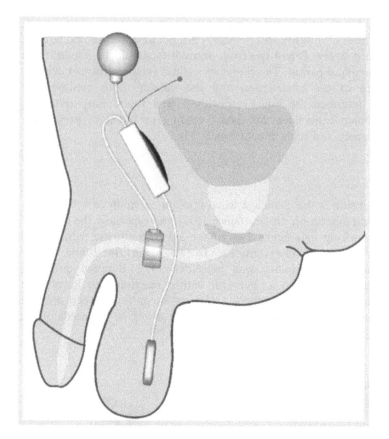

Figure 8   Placement of fine-tuned sensor-controlled artificial sphincter.

Additional Device Handling Instructions

- Passing a catheter (3): before passing a catheter or any other instrument through the urethra, the cuff should be deflated and the device deactivated to prevent potential damage to the AGUS.
- Closed deactivation valve with inflated cuff: the fluid cannot transfer from the cuff to the balloon and sustained outflow obstruction arises. The automatic pressure relief that normally occurs is prevented. Cycling the device can relieve the outflow obstruction.
- Cycling the device is difficult if deactivation occurs when the pump bulb is deflated. If unable to cycle the device, squeezing the sides adjacent to the deactivation button will allow fluid to fill the pump bulb and then the pump can be cycled normally.
- Release of the deactivation valve may require greater pressure than that used to cycle the device.

■ System pressure changes (3) may occur over time if the balloon is filled with radiopaque solution of incorrect concentration.

■ AS 800 and MRI (38): the presence of an AMS 800 prosthesis will not produce harmful effects during scanning. The metallic components were subjected to magnetic field strengths up to 1.5 Tesla without showing unsafe magnetic interaction but they may distort the uniform magnetic field in the vicinity of the implant. The complete compatibility profile within a MRI field has not been established.

CONCLUSION

The AGUS has a definite role in the treatment of urinary incontinence, for adults as well as for children. Overall satisfaction is over 90% (1,30). After 5 years of follow-up 90.4% of patients are well with a working AGUS and 72% required only one operation. The overall reoperation rate is 17%; the expected 5-year product survival rate is 75%.

REFERENCES

1. Petrou SP, Elliott DS, Barrett DM. Artificial urethral sphincter for incontinence. Urology 2000; 56:353–9.
2. Furlow WL. Implantation of a new semiautomatic artificial genitourinary sphincter: experience with primary activation and deactivation in 47 patients. J Urol 1981; 126:741–4.
3. Manual of the AMS Sphincter800Ô Urinary Control System, 1999.
4. AMS Sphincter800Ô, Urinary Prosthesis. Surgical Atlas, 1999.
5. Mark S, Perez LM, Webster GD. Synchronous management of anastomotic contracture and urinary stress incontinence following radical prostatectomy. J Urol 1994; 151:1202–4.
6. Wilson SK, Delk JR II, Henry GD, et al. New surgical Technique for Sphincter urinary control System using upper transverse scrotal Incision. J Urol 2003; 169 (1):261–4.
7. Mottet N, Boyer C, Chartier-Kastler E, et al. Artificial urinary sphincter AMS 800 for urinary incontinence after radical prostatectomy: the French experience. Urol Inter 1998; 60(suppl 2):25–9.
8. Litwiller SE, Kim KB, Fone PD, et al. Post-prostatectomy incontinence and the artificial urinary sphincter: a long-term study of patient satisfaction and criteria for success. J Urol 1996; 156:1975–80.
9. Kowalczyk JJ, Mulcahy JJ. Use of the artificial urinary sphincter in women. Int Urogynecol J 2000; 11:176–9.
10. Duncan HJ, Nurse DE, Mundy AR. Role of the artificial urinary sphincter in the treatment of stress incontinence in women. Br J Urol 1992; 69:141–3.
11. Webster GD, Perez LM, Koury JM, et al. Management of type III urinary stress incontinence using artificial urinary sphincter. Urology 1992; 39:499–503.

12. Costa P, Mottet N, Le Pellec L. Artificial urinary sphincter AMS 800 in operated and unoperated women with Type III incontinence J Urol 19944; 151 (2):477A, abstract 1000.

13. Hadley R, Loisides P, Dickinson M. Long-term follow-up (2–5 years) of transvaginally placed artificial urinary sphincters by an experienced surgeon. J Urol 1996; 153(2):432A, abstract 816.

14. Stone KT, Diokno AC, Mitchell BA. Just how effective is the AMS 800 artificial urinary sphincter? Results of long-term follow-up in females. J Urol 1995; 153(2):433A, abstract 817.

15. Venn SN, Greenwell TJ, Mundy AR. The long-term outcome of artificial urinary sphincters. J Urol 2000; 164:702–7.

16. Gonzalez R, Merino FG, Vaughn M. Long-term results of the artificial urinary sphincter in male patients with neurogenic bladder. J Urol 1995; 154:769–70.

17. Millar EA, Mayo M, Kwan D, et al. Simultaneous augmentation cystoplasty and artificial urinary sphincter placement: infection rates and voiding mechanisms. J Urol 1998; 160:750–2.

18. Strawbridge LR, Kramer SA, Castillo OA, et al. Augmentation cystoplasty and the artificial genitourinary sphincter. J Urol 1989; 142:297–301.

19. Singh G, Thomas DG. Does cystoplasty at the time of an artificial sphincter implantation increase morbidity? (Abstract). Neurourol Urodyn 1994; 13:371.

20. Light JK, Lapin S, Vohra S. Combined use of bowel and the artificial urinary sphincter in reconstruction of the lower urinary tract: infectious complications. J Urol 1005; 153:331–3.

21. Martins FE, Boyd SD. Artificial urinary sphincter in patients following major pelvic surgery and/or radiotherapy: are they less favourable candidates? J Urol 1995; 153:1188–93.

22. Wang Y, Hadley HR. Experiences with the artificial urinary sphincter in the irradiated patient. J Urol 1992; 147:612–3.

23. Perez LM, Webster GD Successful outcome of artificial urinary sphincters in men with post-prostatectomy urinary incontinence despite adverse implantation features. J Urol 1992; 148:1166–70.

24. Gundian JC, Barrett DM, Parulkar BG. Mayo clinic experience with use of the AMS800 artificial urinary sphincter for urinary incontinence following radical prostatectomy. J Urol 1989; 142:1459–61.

25. Marks JL, Light JK. Management of urinary incontinence after prostatectomy with the artificial urinary sphincter. J Urol 1989; 142:302–4.

26. Singh G, Thomas DG. Artificial urinary sphincter for post-prostatectomy incontinence. Br J Urol 1996; 77:248–51.

27. Appell RA. Techniques and results in the implantation of the artificial urinary sphincter in women with Type III urinary stress incontinence by a vaginal approach. Neurourol Urodyn 1988; 7:613–9.

28. Diokno AC, Hollander JB, Alderson TP. Artificial urinary sphincter for recurrent female urinary incontinence: indications and results. J Urol 1987; 138: 778–80.

29. Light JK, Scott FB. Management of urinary incontinence in women with the artificial urinary sphincter. J Urol 1985; 134:476–8.

30. Elliott DS, Barrett DM. Mayo clinic long-term analysis of the functional durability of the AMS 800 artificial urinary sphincter: a review of 323 cases. J Urol 1998; 159:1206–8.
31. Parulkar BG, Barrett DM. Combined implantation of artificial sphincter and penile prosthesis. J Urol 1989; 142:732–5.
32. Scott FB, Fishman IJ, Schotland Y. Experience with simultaneous Implantation of inflatable penile prosthesis and artificial urinary sphincter in 72 patients (Abstract). J Urol 1987; 137:374A.
33. Brito CG, Mulcahy JJ, Mitchell ME, et al. Use of a double cuff AMS800 urinary sphincter for severe stress incontinence. J Urol 1993; 149:283–5.
34. Kowalczyk JJ, Spicer DL, Mulcahy JJ. Long-term Experience with the double-cuff AMS 800 artificial urinary sphincter. Urology 1996; 47:895–7.
35. Fishman IJ. Female incontinence and the artificial urinary sphincter. In: Seidmon EJ, Hanno PM eds. Current Urologic Therapy. 3rd ed. Philadelphia: WB Saunders, 1994:312–5.
36. Fishman IJ, Scott FB. Pregnancy in patients with the artificial urinary sphincter. J Urol 1993; 150:340–1.
37. Schostek S, Ho CN, Wasserman H. Aktorik und Steuerung am Beispiel eines Urologischen Implantats. Biomed Tech 2002; 47(Suppl 1 Pt 2):806–9.
38. Shellock F. MR Procedures and Metallic Objects: Update 1997. Philapdelphia: Lippincott-Raven, 1997:101, 110.

10

Does the Way Hysterectomy Is Performed Make a Difference? How to Prevent Prolapse at the Time of Hysterectomy

Harry Reich

Wyoming Valley Health Care System, Wilkes-Barre, Pennsylvania, and Advanced Laparoscopic Surgeons, Shavertown, Pennsylvania, U.S.A.

Iris Kerin Orbuch

Lenox Hill Hospital and Mount Sinai Medical Center, New York, New York, U.S.A.

Tamer Seckin

Department of Gynecology and Laparoscopy, Kingsbrook Jewish Medical Center, Brooklyn, New York, and Lenox Hill Hospital, New York, New York, U.S.A.

Laparoscopic pelvic floor reconstruction requires a thorough understanding of pelvic floor anatomy. One can undertake reconstructive pelvic surgery only after attaining this knowledge of pelvic floor anatomy. Pelvic organ prolapse is the indication for more than 300,000 surgeries in the United States annually, at a cost of more than one billion dollars (1). The actual incidence of vaginal vault prolapse is unknown but it is thought to occur in 0.1% to 45.0% of patients who have undergone hysterectomy (2,3). Laparoscopic surgery provides excellent visualization, magnification of pelvic structures, reduced hospitalization, decreased pain and recovery time.

It is important to understand that vaginal support comes from interactions between pelvic floor muscles (levator ani) and connective tissue (endopelvic fascia). The levator ani muscles, primarily the iliococcygeus and pubococcygeus muscles, maintain active support of the pelvic floor while the endopelvic fascia and ligaments provide passive support. Operations repair and reconnect breaks in the fascia, the passive support. It was previously thought that stretching of the endopelvic fascia was the primary etiology of prolapse. However it is now thought that a break in the endopelvic fascia results in the prolapse (4).

There is unfortunately no surgical procedure for repair of weakened levator muscles, whose primary etiology is denervation from pudendal nerve injury usually during childbirth. When pelvic floor muscles work properly, there is little strain on the fascial attachments. When muscles fail secondary to trauma or nerve dysfunction, the fascia must assume a supportive role; a role they are not designed for (5). The main goal of any support procedure is to improve function often by restoring anatomy to near its original anatomical position. Laparoscopic surgery aids in visualization and provides magnification of the pelvic floor in order to accomplish this goal. The distention of the pelvis with pneumoperitoneum provides better visualization to aid the surgeon in restoring pelvic anatomy. This chapter reviews pelvic anatomy and various laparoscopic techniques used both to prevent prolapse at the time of hysterectomy and to repair prolapse occurring after hysterectomy (DeLancey Level I support) without using mesh.

ANATOMY

Based on cadaveric dissections Richardson described the vagina as a flattened tube composed of fibro muscular tissue and lined by vaginal epithelium. He states that the anterior wall of the tube is composed of the pubocervicovesicular fascia and the posterior wall of the tube is made of rectovaginal fascia (6).

This connective tissue that envelopes the vagina to its apex is termed endopelvic fascia and is made up of fibroblasts, smooth muscle cells, elastin, and collagen, creating a fibro muscular elastic layer (7). The presacral fascia of the second, third, and fourth sacral vertebrae attaches to uterosacral ligaments. The uterosacral ligaments coalesce with the cardinal ligaments on each side near the pericervical ring. The cardinal ligaments envelope the uterine vessels and fuse with the pericervical ring. This pericervical fascial ring merges with the pubocervical fascia anteriorly and with the rectovaginal fascia posteriorly. Laterally the rectovaginal fascia attaches to the pelvic sidewall. The pubocervicovesicular fascia (the connective tissue at the anterolateral part of the vagina) is attached laterally to the fascia of the obturator internus muscle and creates the arcus tendineus fascia pelvis or "white line". The "white line" originates at the ischial spine and inserts at the pubic bone. Superiorly, the rectovaginal fascia converges with the arcus tendineus half way between the pubic symphysis and ischial spine. Inferiorly, the rectovaginal fascia fuses with the perineal body.

DeLancey describes the principal supports of the vagina and divides pelvic support into three levels. Level I support provides the most superior suspension of the vagina by the cardinal uterosacral complex. Level II support is the lateral support for the upper two thirds of the vagina. Level III provides support to the lower vagina by the fusion of the vagina with perineal membrane and the perineal body.

Level I support, or vertical support, is maintained by superior suspension of the vagina by the cardinal-uterosacral complex. The cardinal-uterosacral complex provides apical support of the upper third of the vagina to the sacrum. The cardinal-uterosacral complex is a mixture of smooth muscle and connective tissue (4). The cardinal ligament is connective tissue that houses the perivascular tissue of the uterine vessels and its constituents are fibrous tissue and nerves (9). The uterosacral ligaments originate from the vertebrae of S2, 3, 4. These ligaments fuse distally and encircle the cervix to form the pericervical ring as they support the upper part of the vagina. Anteriorly the pericervical ring fuses with the pubocervical fascia. Posteriorly, the rectovaginal fascia fuses with the pericervical ring at the level of the ischial spine. Disruption of the cardinal-uterosacral complex results in uterine or vaginal vault prolapse.

An enterocele is defined as a herniation of bowel into the vagina; as a result the pelvic peritoneum gets into direct contact with the vaginal epithelium without any intervening fascia. Richardson divided enteroceles into three types: anterior, apical and posterior based on location of break in the fascia. An *anterior* enterocele occurs when the pubocervical fascia breaks from the cervix or vaginal cuff, and is common in patients with previous sacrospinous ligament suspensions since the vaginal apex is pulled posteriorly. An *apical* enterocele occurs when the pubocervical fascia is separated from the rectovaginal fascia, and is most common in post hysterectomy patients whose pubocervical and rectovaginal fascias are not reapproximated. A posterior enterocele occurs when the rectovaginal fascia detaches from the posterior cervix or vaginal cuff (6).

Level II provides support to the middle third of the vagina, bladder and rectum. As mentioned previously, anterior vaginal support is provided by the pubocervicovesicular fascia and posterior support is provided by rectovaginal fascia. The pubocervicovesicular fascia is attached at the sidewall to the arcus tendineus fascia of the pelvis and the medial fascia of the levator ani. These structures form a horizontal support sheet. When the endopelvic fascia breaks off from the pelvic sidewall a paravaginal cystocele is formed.

Level III support occurs as the pubocervical fascia fuses with the perineal membrane and the rectovaginal fascia fuses with the perineal membrane. Below the level of the levator ani, the perineal membrane is found. The main function of level III support is to preserve the vaginal outlet and preclude any level I or II defects from falling below the levator plate (5).

The muscular support comes from the pelvic diaphragm or the levator ani. Of the levator ani muscles, the ilicoccygeus and pubococcygeus provide the majority of support. The iliococcygeus muscle comes from the tendious arch of the levator ani muscle and inserts between the anus and coccyx. The pubococcygeus muscles start on the inner aspect of the pubic bone and traverse to insert onto the sacrum. These two muscles maintain active support. The levator ani muscles are usually damaged from childbirth secondary to pudendal nerve injury. Damage can also occur as a result of chronic constipation, chronic lung problems or anything that increases intra-abdominal pressure. After these muscles are damaged the endopelvic fascia takes over as the primary pelvic support (10).

LAPAROSCOPIC TECHNIQUES FOR LEVEL I SUPPORT

Laparoscopic vault suspension to restore Level I support can be attained by either the laparoscopic uterosacral ligament suspension or by laparoscopic sacral colpopexy. Sacral colpopexy usually requires the use of mesh. HR abandoned its use in 1993 after a single case of mesh cuff erosion 10 years after sacral colpopexy by laparotomy. We prefer not using mesh.

Reich advocates laparoscopic uterosacral ligament suspension as part of every total laparoscopic hysterectomy to prevent future prolapse. Mesh is never used. The evolution from McCall's original culdeplasty to its laparoscopic counterpart will be described, including methods to lessen the effects of a high cystocele on urinary retention. Also included are laparoscopic techniques to repair prolapse occurring after hysterectomy without the use of mesh.

McCall Culdeplasty

In 1957 McCall described repair of an enterocele at the time of vaginal hysterectomy. McCall reported on forty-five patients in his landmark paper and described no recurrence of enterocele. His technique described using *internal* and *external* sutures. The *internal* sutures are nonabsorbable (described as silk, cotton, or linen) to obliterate the enterocele sac by taking bites of both uterosacrals and posterior peritoneum. More specifically, his first suture takes the left uterosacral ligament, then the enterocele sac "at intervals of 1 to 2 cm" until the right uterosacral ligament is reached and the suture passed through it. This suture is left untied to help guide more similarly placed sutures above the first suture. The number of internal sutures depends on the size of the enterocele sac. These *internal* sutures are not tied until the *external* sutures are placed. Three *external* sutures are then placed. McCall inserted a "No. 1 catgut suture from the vaginal side just right of the midline of the vagina about 2 cm above its posterior cut edge." Next the right uterosacral is taken, followed by the left uterosacral and out the vaginal wall at the same level as this suture was entered, but just left of the midline. The suture is not tied. Two more sutures are placed, each higher than the last. The top suture brings the vault to its highest level. Next the internal sutures and then the external sutures are tied. The peritoneum is closed in the usual fashion. McCall stated that his method maintains vaginal length and does not narrow the vault as it obliterates the cul-de-sac (11, 12).

There have been several modifications to McCall's original technique. The Mayo Clinic version, pioneered by Richard Symmonds, described a modified endopelvic fascia repair. A wedge of vaginal epithelium is excised from both the anterior and posterior wall to allow access to the lateral vaginal supports. After the enterocele is excised, one to three *internal* McCall sutures are placed. Next, external sutures are placed incorporating the posterior vaginal wall, cul-de-sac peritoneum, paravaginal and para-rectal tissue, and uterosacral-cardinal ligament complex. More external sutures can be placed based on the length of the vault (13–14).

Cruikshank and Kovac showed in a prospective clinical trial that a modified McCall culdeplasty that reattaches the uterosacral ligaments to the apex of the vaginal is very effective at preventing future apical defects. At three years, the incidence of apical defects in the McCall group was 6% *versus* 30% in the control group (15).

These techniques addressed posterior vaginal wall support, but failed to mention the frequently occurring high cystocele in the anterior vaginal wall that often results in urinary retention.

Laparoscopic Operations

The McCall culdeplasty is a vaginal procedure. (By today's terminology, culdeplasty is colpoplasty or culdoplasty. Colpoplasty is done vaginally and culdoplasty is done from above.) It was applied through an abdominal incision by Thomas Elkins with good results. Early experience with a total laparoscopic approach to hysterectomy was accompanied by various methods of cuff closure. These can be simplified into the traditional transverse cuff closure and the vertical cuff closure. The transverse closure is accompanied usually by uterosacral ligament suspension on each side. The vertical closure almost always is done with a McCall type stitch, bringing the uterosacral ligaments together across the midline. We call this laparoscopic vertical closure a laparoscopic high McCall culdeplasty (LHM).

Reich adapted the McCall culdeplasty to total laparoscopic hyster-ectomy after listening to a lecture on "abdominal incision high McCall" by Thomas Elkins in 1992 (17). This technique addressed posterior vaginal wall and vault support, but failed to mention the frequently occurring high cystocele in the anterior vaginal wall that often results in urinary retention. By 1994, the high McCall technique had undergone major modifications by Reich to include the anterior vagina.

He identifies four different laparoscopic operations using this technique or its modifications. The first two are done at the time of hysterectomy and the others are for post hysterectomy vaginal cuff prolapse or possible cuff pathology, especially pain:

1. prophylactic technique to prevent prolapse at time of hysterectomy (LHM),
2. repair of prolapse or occult prolapse with urinary retention (high cystocele) at time of hysterectomy (Reich modification of HM),
3. repair of vaginal cuff prolapse after hysterectomy (Reich modification of HM),
4. operation for post hysterectomy pelvic pain and/or dyspareunia by excision of vaginal cuff scar (endometriosis or fibronodular cuff adhesions) followed by vaginal apical elevation onto uterosacral ligaments (Reich modification of HM).

Laparoscopic Technique at the Time of Hysterectomy (TLH) to Prevent Future Prolapse

This procedure is indicated when minimal or no prolapse is evident and the patient has no urinary complaints, especially retention related. It is considered a part of every total laparoscopic hysterectomy.

After the uterus has been removed, the vagina is occluded to maintain pneumoperitoneum during closure of the vaginal cuff. The uterosacral ligaments are identified usually from the white markings from bipolar desiccation and/or with the aid of a rectal probe. The left uterosacral ligament is elevated, and a 0-Vicryl suture on a CT-1 needle is placed through it using an oblique Cook needle holder. The suture is then placed through the left cardinal ligament, located at the left posterolateral vagina just below the uterine vessels, then through the rectovaginal fascia and posterior peritoneum parallel to the cut edge of the posterior vaginal epithelium, and then to and through the right posterolateral vagina and cardinal ligament to the right uterosacral ligament. This suture is tied extracorporeally and provides excellent support to the vaginal cuff apex, elevating it superiorly and posteriorly toward the hollow of the sacrum. The rest of the vagina and its overlying pubocervicovesicular fascia are closed vertically with one or two 0-Vicryl interrupted sutures. In most cases the peritoneum is not closed (Figs. 1–3).

Cystoscopy is routinely done after vaginal closure to assure ureteral patency, 10 minutes after intravenous administration of one ampule of Indigo Carmine dye. This is especially necessary when the ureter is identified but not dissected. Efflux of blue dye should be visualized through both ureteral orifices. The bladder wall should also be inspected for suture and thermal defects.

This technique for vaginal vault closure at the time of TLH has been used by Reich in all cases over the last 18 years, and no cuff prolapses have come to his attention.

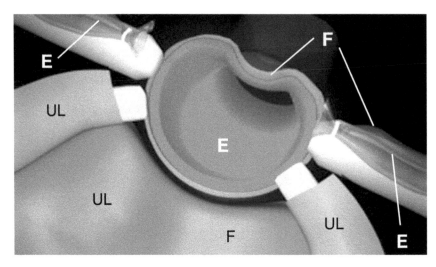

Figure 1 Panoramic view of the pelvis after hysterectomy, cervicectomy, or after excision of vaginal cuff scar. The uterosacral ligaments (UL) appear pink and fleshy, the cardinal ligaments enclose the uterine vessels, the rectovaginal fascia of the posterior vaginal cuff and the pubocervicovesicular fascia are labeled F; the vaginal epithelium is labeled E.

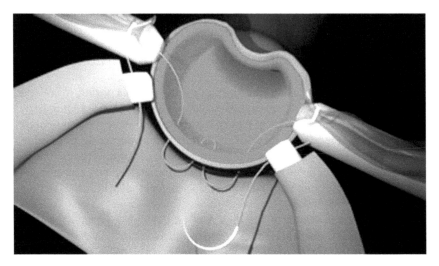

Figure 2 Panoramic view after the placement of the first suture on a CT-1 needle before tying. This first suture has been placed through the left uterosacral ligament, the left cardinal ligament below the uterine vessels, the rectovaginal fascia of the posterior vaginal cuff (two bites), the right cardinal ligament, and the right uterosacral ligament.

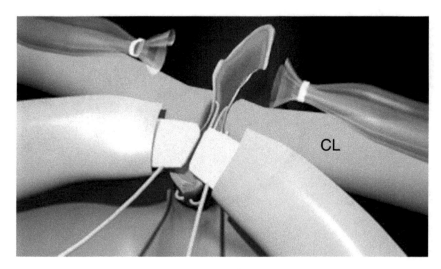

Figure 3 The first suture is completed. Note the plication of the uterosacral ligaments and the cardinal ligaments (CL) to the posterior vagina/rectovaginal fascia bringing both uterosacral ligaments and rectovaginal fascia together in the midline.

Repair of Prolapse or Occult Prolapse with Urinary Retention (High Cystocele) at total Laparoscopic Hysterectomy

Following TLH with the above described cuff closure, Reich observes that many patients give an unsolicited description of improvement in micturition at their post-operative visit. This may be because urinary retention present from a high cystocele adjacent to the cervix is reduced by TLH with routine cuff vertical suspension.

The technique to be described not only addresses the posterior wall, but the anterior wall as well. Uterovaginal prolapse may be obvious. Alternately, urinary retention may be present from a high cystocele adjacent to the cervix.

Unfortunately, the symptoms of urinary retention are seldom volunteered by the patient seeking hysterectomy and should be ascertained by the physician during the history. The simple question is "Do you feel like you are completely emptying your bladder or do you feel that you still have to go after urinating?"

Reich's modification of the high McCall culdeplasty brings the anterior vagina much higher than the posterior wall. This procedure can be done during the same surgery as hysterectomy or for prolapse after a previous hysterectomy. After the "high McCall" suspension first suture brings the uterosacral and cardinal ligaments and posterior vagina together in the midline, subsequent sutures bring the lateral and anterior vagina with overlying pubocervicovesicular fascia onto the uterosacral ligaments working progressively towards the sacrum.

At the time of hysterectomy, after the uterus is removed, a vaginal device or probe is placed in the vagina to maintain pneumoperitoneum. Vaginal hemostasis is obtained using microbipolar forceps until complete, so as to not be dependent on compression by sutures. The left uterosacral ligament and posterolateral vagina are elevated. Going from left to right, the same 0-Vicryl suture is placed through the left uterosacral ligament, then through the left cardinal ligament followed by posterior vaginal tissue including the rectovaginal fascia but minimal vaginal epithelium. The suture exits near the midline then back through rectovaginal fascia and vagina on the right followed by the right cardinal ligament and right uterosacral ligament. Extracorporeal knot tying is done, pulling up the vaginal apex and elevating it both posteriorly and superiorly toward the hollow of the sacrum. The first suture is placed below the level of the uterine artery pedicle as the cardinal ligament is identified as the thick band of connective tissue beneath the ligated uterine vessels.

The second suture is placed through the uterosacral ligaments closer to the sacrum and then through the endopelvic fascia just above the uterine vessel pedicle (Figs. 4 and 5). The third suture is placed through the uterosacral

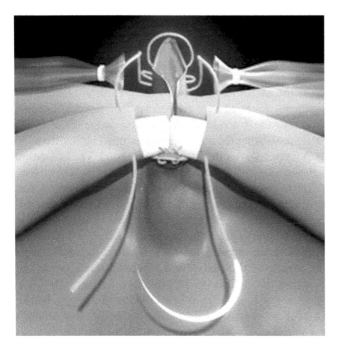

Figure 4 A second 0-Ethibond suture is placed through the left uterosacral ligament, the left cardinal ligament above the uterine vessels, the pubocervicov-esicular fascia of the anterior vaginal cuff across to the right cardinal ligament above the uterine vessels, and the right uterosacral ligament closer to the sacrum.

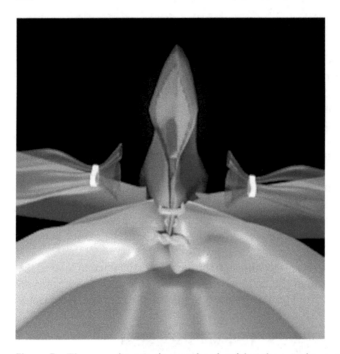

Figure 5 The second suture is completed, raising the anterior vaginal cuff above the posterior vagina.

ligaments even closer to the sacrum and through the endopelvic fascia well above the cardinal ligament, resulting in a vertical vaginal closure. The last suture is usually placed into the anterior vagina/pubocervicovesicular fascia above the cuff at 12 o'clock to bring the anterior vagina much higher than the posterior wall (Fig. 6). All sutures after the first are 0-Ethibond. The last suture also is placed at the highest level toward the sacral area. As with any suspension, special care must be taken to ensure the integrity of the rectum and ureters. The sutures must not constrict the rectum, which is identified throughout the procedure with a rectal probe inside it. This suspension achieves a physiologic position of the vagina. In addition, it provides the vagina with good depth since the vagina can go high towards the sacral region where the uterosacral ligaments originate (Fig. 7). The closure of the vagina in a vertical fashion avoids the ureters, as the sutures stay in the midline (17,18,19).

Uterosacral ligaments are sometimes identified and tagged before TLH by putting the uterus on upward tension into an anteverted/anteflexed position and placing a Vicryl gathering suture around them near their sacral portion. These sutures can be left long to aid those surgeons more comfortable doing a laparoscopic assisted vaginal hysterectomy (LAVH) instead of a TLH. During LAVH, the suture can be pulled out through the vagina with a finger and used with a free needle to attach the vaginal vault apex to

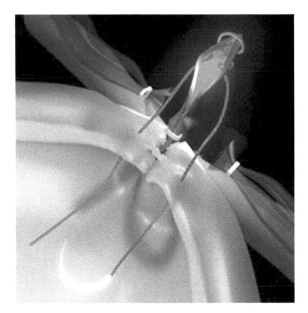

Figure 6   The uterosacral ligaments near the sacral promontory are sutured to the pubocervicovesicular fascia and the anterior vagina at a higher level.

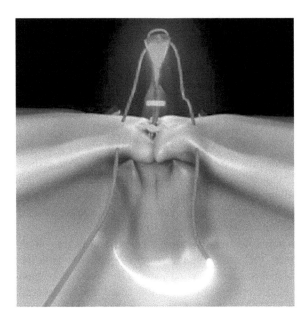

Figure 7   The uterosacral ligaments near the sacral promontory are sutured to the pubocervicovesicular fascia and the anterior vagina at a still higher level and above the anterior limit of the vaginal cuff.

the uterosacral ligaments at a much higher level than is safe using a purely vaginal approach (Fig. 8).

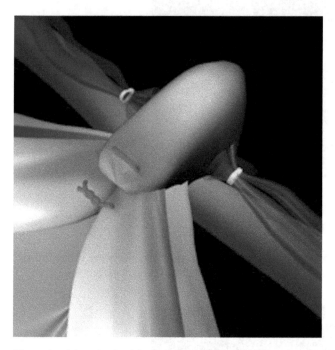

Figure 8   After the final knot is completed, excellent support of the anterior vagina and its fascia is seen elevated to near the sacral promontory. High cystocele has been reduced.

Repair of Vaginal Cuff Prolapse after Hysterectomy

Vaginal vault prolapse can usually be repaired by the technique described above. Again, the anterior vaginal wall is elevated higher than the original posterior wall. In almost all cases, the detached uterosacral ligament can be identified far from the vaginal cuff apex scar early in the operation and isolated with a gathering stitch.

Laparoscopic uterosacral ligament vault suspension begins with identifying the vaginal apex, the proximal uterosacral ligaments and the ureters. The surgeon should check for an enterocele. The ureter may pass near an enterocele sac; thus, the ureters should be identified and uncovered by incising the peritoneum medial to them. A vaginal probe is inserted and is pushed towards the patient's head. An enterocele sac, which is composed of peritoneum and vaginal epithelium, can be visualized as a thin translucent membrane. The peritoneum over the vaginal apex is incised or excised so that the pubocervical fascia can be seen anteriorly and laterally and the rectovaginal fascia posteriorly. If the enterocele is large, the redundant peritoneum should be excised. A rectal probe can be placed and pushed in a direction away from the vaginal probe. This helps better visualization of the rectovaginal septum and allows better access to the rectovaginal fascia. Next, the pubocervical and rectovaginal fascia are reapproximated vertically with absorbable suture to restore the fibro-muscular tube. With the rectal probe in place, the uterosacral ligaments can be traced to near the sacrum. Next, using a nonabsorbable suture, such as Ethibond on a curved needle, a bite of the proximal part of the uterosacral ligament is taken. Next, a bite through the ipsilateral recto-vaginal fascia and the corresponding pubocervical fascia is taken. Finally, the contralateral pubocervical/rectovaginal fascia and the proximal con-tralateral uterosacral ligament are secured with the same suture. Extracorporeal knot tying is used to suspend the vault to the uterosacral ligaments across the midline (19,20).

Post-Hysterectomy Excision of Vaginal Cuff Scar (Endometriosis or Adhesions) Followed by Elevation onto Uterosacral Ligaments for Pain and/or Dyspareunia (Reich Modification of HM)

Some patients present with pain and discomfort without obvious prolapse. If the fibrotic cuff is excised, the defect repaired with interrupted vertical sutures, and elevated onto the uterosacral ligaments across the midline, many of these patients will experience relief of pain. The exact mechanism is unclear.

CONCLUSION

There are many different methods to address vaginal vault prolapse and reduce its incidence at the time of hysterectomy and thereafter. Whichever method is employed, it is important to use the principles of anatomy to guide reconstruction. In order to repair prolapse, the pubocervical and rectovaginal fascia must be reapproximated to each other and to the car-dinal-uterosacral complex at the level of the ischial spine, ideally at the time of hysterectomy. Reich's adaptation of the vaginal McCall culdoplasty addresses both the posterior and anterior wall near the vaginal apex. It brings the anterior vagina higher than the posterior wall. Mesh is not used with this approach to minimize rejection and all the shortcomings of mesh. He does not believe that mesh should be used during laparoscopic or laparotomy hysterectomy for conditions other than frank prolapse. And even in those cases, other techniques that avoid mesh should be considered.

Although this chapter only addresses Level I DeLancey support pro-cedures, it is important to understand that other compartment defects may coexist. (Level I support provides the most superior suspension of the vagina by the cardinal-uterosacral complex.) We understand but do not support the philosophy of Wattiez et al. that a global approach to pelvic reconstruction be instituted. [As multiple compartment defects may coexist, it is important to repair all the pelvic floor defects in the same operation (21,22).] But the future of mesh remains to be determined, and time and reimbursement issues for multiple procedures during the same operation will limit this approach in the immediate future, at least in the United States.

REFERENCES

1. Subak LL, Waetjen LE, van den Eeden S, Thom DH, Vittinghoff E, Brown JS. Cost of pelvic organ prolapse surgery in the United States. Obstet Gynecol 2001; 98:646–51.
2. Cruikshank SH. Sacrospinous fixation—should this be performed at the time of vaginal hysterectomy? Am J Obstet Gynecol 1991; 164:1073–76.
3. Karram M, Goldwasser S, Kleeman S, Steele A, Vassallo B, Walsh P. High uterosacral vaginal vault suspension with fascial reconstruction for vaginal repair of enterocele and vaginal vault prolapse. Am J Obstet Gynecol 2001; 185: 1339–1342.
4. DeLancey JO, Richardson AC. Anatomy of Genital Support. In Urogynecologic Surgery. Maryland: Aspen Publishers, Ch 3, 1992:19–33.
5. Fleischmann NB, Nitti VW. Pelvic floor reconstruction: state-of-the-art and beyond. Urol Clin N Am 2004; 31:757–67.
6. Richardson AC. Anatomic Defects in Rectocele and Enterocele. J Pelvic Surg 1995; 1,4:214–21.
7. Strohbehn K. Normal pelvic floor anatomy. Obstet Gynecol Clin North Am 1998; 25:683–705.
8. Cundiff GW, Fenner D. Evaluation and treatment of women with rectocele: focus on associated defecatory and sexual dysfunction. Obstet Gynecol 2004; 104(6):1403–21.
9. Campbell RM. The anatomy and histology of the sacrouterine ligaments. Am J Obstet Gynecol 1950; 59:1–12.
10. Liu CY. Laparoscopic pelvic reconstructive surgery: Part 1. ObGyn News 2004; 39(19):58–9.
11. McCall ML. Posterior Culdoplasty. Surgical correction of enterocele during vaginal hysterectomy; a preliminary report. Obstet Gyn 1957; 10(6):595–602.
12. Karram MM, Kleeman SD. Vaginal vault prolapse. In: Te Linde's Operative Gynecology. 9th ed. Philadephia: Lipincott Williams & Wilkins, 2003: 999–1020.
13. Symmonds RE, Pratt JH. Vaginalprolapse following hysterectomy. Am J Obstet Gyn 1960; 79(5):899–909.
14. Symmonds RE, Williams TJ, Lee RA, Webb MJ. Posthysterectomy enterocele and vaginal vault prolapse Am J Obstet Gyn 1981; 140(8):852–9.
15. Lee Al, Symmondds RE. Surgical repair of posthysterectomy vault prolapse. Am J Obstet Gyn 1972; 112:953–6.

16. Cruishank SH, Kovac SR. Randomized comparison of three surgical methods used at the time of vaginal hysterectomy to prevent posterior enterocele. Am J Obstet Gynecol 1999; 180:953–865.
17. Reich H, McGlynn F, Sekel L. Total laparoscopic hysterectomy. Gynaecol Endosc 1993; 2:59–63.
18. Liu CY, Reich H. Correction of genital prolapse. J Endourol 1996; 10,3:259–65.
19. Reich H, Vancaillie TG. Recent advances in laparoscopic hysterectomy and pelvic floor reconstruction. Surgical Technology International III. (International Developments in Surgery and Surgical Research), San Francisco, CA: Universal Press, 1995.
20. Liu CY. Laparoscopic Pelvic Reconstructive surgery: Part 2. ObGyn News 2004; 39(21):42–3.
21. Miklos JR, Moore RD, Kohli N. Laparoscopic pelvic floor repair. Obstet Gynecol Clin N Am 2004; 31:551–65.
22. Wattiez A, Mashiah R, Donoso M. Laparoscopic repair of vaginal vault prolapse. Curr Opin Obstet Gynecol 2003; 15:315–19.

11

Vaginal Vault Prolapse: Treatment of Posterior IVS

Peter von Theobald

Department of Obstetrics, Gynecology, and Reproductive Medicine,
University Hospital of Caen, Caen, France

INTRODUCTION

The use of prostheses aimed to be interposed between the organs can be justified by the number of recurrences after classical vaginal surgery. The recurrences are caused by the fact that in patients suffering from descent, there has been a decrease in the quality of the perineal collagen. The simple mechanical restoration of the tension in the fascial structures therefore does not result in a durable effect over time. Classical promonto-fixation (1) followed by the laparoscopic technique (2–5) allows for the use of synthetic materials instead of a patient's fascia and therefore obtains a more durable anatomical result. The invasiveness of the laparotomic approach on the one hand and the difficulty of the promonto-fixation using the laparoscopic approach on the other could well offer a predominant place in the treatment of female pelvic organ prolapse to a vaginal technique, in which prostheses can be placed without risks or difficulties in the same spaces used by the other techniques.

Prostheses of polypropylene have been used through the vaginal approach for urinary stress incontinence (USI) for well over five years, proving their excellent biocompatibility. The percentage of infection and erosion through the mucosa due to infection are very low. Other materials, such as prostheses covered by collagen of porcine or bovine origin, seem very promising.

The interposition of prostheses between the organs has to fulfill different criteria: the prostheses should not move and these should allow for movement of the different organs (bladder, vagina, and rectum) and respect the suppleness of the walls. A too-rigid fixation should be avoided. The aim is to generate strong and durable collagen at the specific sites; one could call it a surgical-directed cicatrization: "bio-engineering."

The triple perineal operation with prostheses (T-POP) is aimed to respond to these requisites by inserting three prostheses of polypropylene (Fig. 1). The authors describe a variation of the technique with conservation of the uterus. Historically, a vaginal hysterectomy has been performed during the treatment of genital descent. The start of the laparotomic and later laparoscopic techniques for promontory fixation has engendered a change in the radical move toward a more conservative approach leaving the uterus in situ. In doing so there has been a reduction in postoperative morbidity and postoperative pain. It seems obvious that a uterine weight of 100 g in a postmenopausal patient is not able to influence the outcome of a treatment for prolapse. It is also clear that a possible future operation at the level of the uterus, i.e., in the case of myoma formation or cancer, is not hampered by the operation for descent. Although still a matter of debate, the authors preserve the uterus in all cases where there is no obvious reason to remove it (cervical dystrophy, multiple fibroids, or abnormal uterine bleeding episode not responding to medical treatment).

The anterior prosthesis treats the cystocele. Its anterior extremity is passed through a dissection plane, allowing for a close contact with the posterior face of the pubic bone (the space of Retzius). The posterior extremity is fixed to the isthmus of the uterus, closing the path for the

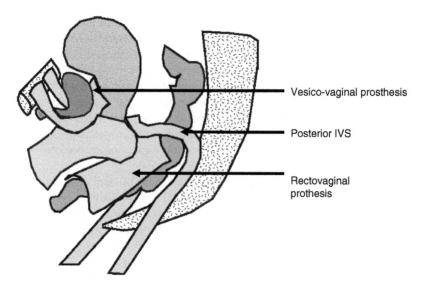

Vesico-vaginal prosthesis

Posterior IVS

Rectovaginal prothesis

Figure 1   The triple perineal operation with prosthesis.

descent of the cystocele as described in the standard work of Forthergill. The posterior intravaginal slingplasty (IVS), or trans-levator mesh, treats the uterine descent, the enterocele and the rectocele occurring above the levator muscle. This prosthesis constitutes the vault of the repair in the case of a three compartment prolapse. This prosthesis permits to elevate the vaginal posterior cul de sac backwards and aim it toward the sacrum in the direction of S3. In doing this, the technique becomes an alternative for the Richter spino-fixation and the promontory-fixation techniques.

The posterior prosthesis deals with the rectocele. This mesh is connected at the high end to the posterior IVS and at the lower end to the perineal body on both sides of the anus.

This technique perfectly fits the definition of a repair without tension within the principles of the integral repair theory. The technique can also be used to treat urinary stress incontinence (USI) adding a sub-urethral sling passing through the vaginal mucosa. Here, a separate incision is made to avoid the movement of the prosthesis toward the bladder neck.

SURGICAL TECHNIQUE

The first incision is an anterior and sagittal colpotomy. If the surgeon foresees the placement of a sub-urethral, retro pubic, prosthesis for the treatment of USI, the colpotomy has to stop some 4 cm from the meatus urethrae externus. This leaves enough space to be able to perform a separate incision for this mesh. When both prostheses are placed within the same longer incision, the risk exists for the sub-urethral mesh to slip towards the bladder neck in a later stage in time.

The dissection of the vesico vaginal and the vesico uterine spaces has to be wide. On the lateral side, the dissection finishes at the pelvic fascia. This fascia has to be perforated on both sides of the bladder neck. Here, a tunnel is opened towards the space of Retzius.

The anterior prosthesis, designated to be placed between the vagina and the bladder is 4 cm wide and made out of polypropylene. The average length is of 6 to 8 cm. Two 1 cm by 3 cm arms extend from the anterior end of the mesh. The prosthesis is cut out of a sheet of 15×8 cm. This leaves enough material to also produce the posterior prosthesis.

If the cystocele is very large or if the vagina is very deep, 1 or 2 cm are added to the average length making the prosthesis 7 to 9 cm long. The aim is to support the bladder from the pubis to the uterine isthmus.

The two anterior extensions are brought through the tunnels in the pelvic fascia and are placed flat on the posterior aspect of the symphysis pubis. To accomplish this maneuver the index finger or a dissection forceps, without teeth is used. The adhesion to the posterior aspect of the symphysis pubis is enough to guarantee a reliable and strong anterior anchoring of the prosthesis. A variation to the technique is the lateral fixation using the trans-obturator route. Two reabsorbable sutures are used to fix the other, deeper end of the anterior prosthesis to the uterine isthmus. If the uterus is absent, this part of the mesh can be fixed to the vaginal vault, the uterine sacral ligaments or to the trans-levator prosthesis (IVS posterior).

To the lateral aspect it is possible to attach the prosthesis to the arcus tendineus of the levator ani muscle (ileo coccygeus). This technique is used if the cystocele is very important.

It is very important to avoid folding of the prosthesis as well as sharp crest in the prosthesis as much as possible. The prosthesis has to be left as flat as possible. The other aspect is the absence of tension.

An anterior colpography is performed with a fast resorbable suture. The suture goes through vaginal mucosa and fascia. It is important not to perform a colpotomy. The colpotomy at the end of the procedures gives a more satisfying image by bringing the structures back under tension. In the longer run, however, the colpotomy causes a reduction in thickness of the vaginal mucosa and fascia.

The repair of the fascia with the prosthesis genders the treatment of the cystocele. The prosthesis also brings the vagina back into its original axis. The vagina, consisting of very vital tissues will bring itself back under tension just a few days after the procedure and will adhere to the level of the dissection and to the prosthesis. This guarantees its normal length and normal thickness of the walls.

A classical posterior colpotomy is performed taking care not to incise the perineum. The latter maneuver avoids excessive pain sensation with the patient. The deepest point of the incision reaches the uterine cervix. The recto-vaginal septum and the enterocele are dissected out. The two para-rectal fossae are opened by the fingers and sharp dissection with scissors if needed. The landmarks on both sides are the ischial spines, the sacro-spinal ligaments and the muscle bundles of the levator ani muscles ileo- and pubo-coccygeus muscles). On the anterior side the uterine isthmus is exposed at the insertion of the sacro-uterine ligaments. This is a classical dissection and is carried out without valves. The complications are the same as in classical surgery: rectal injuries—especially in case of re-intervention—bleeding and secondary haematomas. The dissection therefore has to be very cautious and meticulous as it is the cornerstone of the future results of the repair of the rectocele by the prosthesis.

An incision is made some 3 cm outside and posterior on both sides of the anal margin. This is a safe area because at a distance from the vascular and nerve bundles, some starting at the foramen ischiadicum and running at 3 o'clock and 9 o'clock and some coming from the coccyx at 6 o'clock, that converge to the anus. This incision allows for a straight penetration, in the horizontal line, into the ischio-rectal space. The tunnelizer is inserted through the incision in the gluteus into the ischio-rectal space (Figs. 2 and 3). The instrument is kept away from the rectum by the levator ani muscles

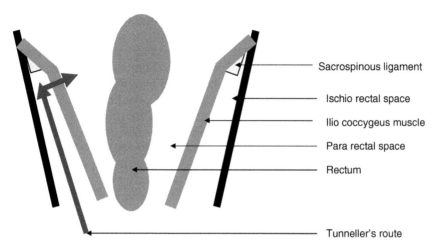

Sacrospinous ligament

Ischio rectal space

Ilio coccygeus muscle

Para rectal space

Rectum

Tunneller's route

Figure 2 Trajectory of the IVS tunneller (*frontal view*).

and by the finger of the physician that is placed into the para rectal fossa. Under tactile control of the finger, the smooth end of the instrument is pushed alongside the muscle plate until it reaches the sacro-spinal ligament some 2 cm inside the ischiadic spine. At this level the smooth end of the instrument is allowed to perforate the muscle plate to enter into contact with the palpating finger. This maneuver allows for the tunnelizer to be prevented from entering the rectum and to be brought outside the colpotomy opening. The polypropylene prosthesis is pouched through the tunnelizer with a plastic trocar.

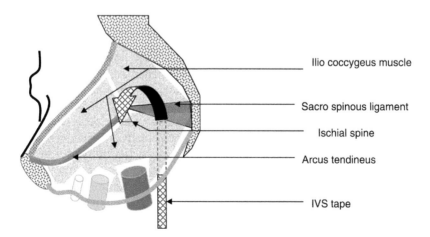

Ilio coccygeus muscle

Sacro spinous ligament

Ischial spine

Arcus tendineus

IVS tape

Figure 3 Trajectory of the IVS tunneller (para median sagittal view).

Once the prosthesis is in place, the tunnelizer is withdrawn. It is mandatory that the mesh has sufficient tissue contact. If manual traction on the mesh does not gender any kind of resistance, the mesh should be withdrawn and repositioned deeper in the levator muscle. The position of the opening in the muscle should be checked thoroughly; it has to be located in the middle of the muscle at the contact with the ischio-sacral ligament. The prosthesis is fixed to the utero-sacral ligaments, the isthmus of the uterus, and the vaginal vault by two resorbable stitch. The aim here is to treat the uterine descent, the enterocele, the vaginal vault prolapse, and the rectocele above the musculus levator.

The prosthesis that is brought in between the rectum and the vagina, on an average, measures 8 cm in length and 4 cm in width. The edges are smooth and rounded, as are those of the anterior prosthesis. The aim here is to fill the rectovaginal septum and in doing so to reinforce it to treat the rectocele. On the high distal end, this prosthesis is fixed to the posterior IVS prosthesis with two resorbable stitches. The lower proximal end is fixed to the perineal body on both sides of the anus with two resorbable stitches. This prosthesis has to be maneuvered so that it lies flat on the rectum. When the system is brought under tension it will be hauled towards the concave face of the sacrum together with the vaginal vault, the uterus, and the vesico-vaginal prosthesis that is attached to the uterine isthmus. No colpotomy is performed. It is recommended to close the anterior colpotomy with a running resorbable stitche before putting tension on the two lateral extremities of the posterior IVS; after hauling the system into place, the posterior vaginal culde-sac will be far from the vulvar opening, making suturing of the colpotomy difficult.

A mesh is pressed into the vagina, to be removed after 24 hr to assure approximation between the vaginal walls and the prostheses and to compress the cleavage planes. A stay catheter is left in the bladder also for 24 hr.

MATERIALS AND METHODS

One hundred consecutive patients have been operated with this technique between June 2001 and December 2002. All the patients have been scored using the POP-Q (6) classification. All patients did have a urodynamic assessment before the surgery. Twenty-one patients who suffered from severe dyschesia did undergo an anorectal evaluation that incorporated a defecography and an anal manometry. Ten of the patients did present with a rectocele under the level of the musculus levator ani and intussusception. Thirty-seven patients did have prior abdominal surgery for organ prolapse (one to four operations by abdominal and/or vaginal route). Of this last category of patients, 25 did have a hysterectomy and 17 a myography of the levator muscles with a posterior colpography. All of the patients did present with an indication for IVS posterior. The main symptom in 18 patients was an isolated vaginal vault prolapse. Twenty patients presented with vaginal vault prolapse or uterine descent combined with a rectocele. Sixty two patients had three compartment organ prolapse. USI or a closure pressure of <30 cm of water at urodynamic examination was present in 48 patients.

All per- and post-operative complication have been registered. Post-operative checks have been planned at six weeks post-operatively, six months for a second follow-up visit and thereafter on a yearly basis.

RESULTS

The median age of the patients is of 60 years (36–82). The follow-up visits range from 6 to 42 months (median of 19 months). IVS posterior has been the sole method of treatment in 18 patients. In 20 patients, a supplementary prosthesis has been placed between the rectum and the vaginal and fixed to the posterior IVS. In 62 patients, the full Triple Perineal Operation with prostheses has been performed. In 15 of the 75 patients still having a uterus in situ, a hysterectomy has been performed where there existed an indication for hysterectomy. In 48 patients, a treatment for USI has been performed, at the time of the main surgery, using a sub-urethral prosthesis (anterior IVS).

The median duration for the interventions was of 58 min (40 min when no hysterectomy was associated, 65 when a hysterectomy or an anterior IVS was associated).

Eight preoperative complications have been documented: seven bladder injuries at the time of entering the space of Retzius and one bleeding out of the space of Retzius treated with compression. One injury to the rectum has been seen during the dissection in a patient with several previous surgeries. This opening in the rectum of 5 mm have been detected just above the anal sphincter and treated with closing and covered by bringing the levator muscles over the rectum with absorbable sutures. The posterior IVS could still be placed as this lesion was situated a distance from the posterior vaginal cul de sac.

Five patients had a hemoglobin fall to 10 g Hb after the surgery. Six patients have been lost to follow-up. The postoperative complications are listed in Table 1.

Hospital stay ranged between 2 and 10 days (median of four days). Functional and anatomical results are listed in Table 2.

DISCUSSION

The three erosions of the anterior and the posterior vaginal wall have been treated by partial excision of the protruding prosthesis and closure of the vaginal mucosa.

Table 1   Postoperative Complications

Early			
Fever > 38°C	5		
Urinary tract infections	6		
Hematoma space of Retzius	2	Observation by means of ultrasound	
Late			
Erosions	3	Three anterior after 2 and 18 months	Excision of the eroded part and simple suture
Infection	2	Posterior after 15 days (infected hematoma) and five months (infected erosion)	Complete removal of the prosthesis

The fourth erosion caused by a rectovaginal prosthesis, has been diagnosed late and recurred after partial excision and closure. Here, the complete removal of the prosthesis became mandatory because of infection. The para-rectal hematoma was diagnosed six days after dismissal of the patient out of the hospital and was drained by a posterior colpotomy. High fever did set in, followed by a purulent discharge made removal of the recto vaginal prosthesis and the posterior IVS necessary on the postoperative 11th day. The uninfected vesico-vaginal prosthesis was left in place. The second surgery was uneventful. The patient recovered fully and quickly antibiotic coverage.

Table 2   Anatomical and Functional Results (*n* = 92 Patients)

Cystocele repair (62 anterior prostheses)	Eight failures after six weeks (insufficient correction)	Three secondary failures
Rectocele repair (82 posterior prostheses)	No failures after six weeks (insufficient correction)	One failure after six months
Vaginal vault repair (92 posterior IVS)	No failures after six weeks (insufficient correction)	One failure after one year
USI treatment (48 anterior IVS)	Zero in this group, four in the group without anterior IVS	11 dysuria (transient)
Pain	One dysparaeunia, three perineal pain > at six months	
Transit	Two de novo constipations, six improvement of mechanical dyschesia	

One of the patients did complain of secondary dysparoenia six months postoperatively. The right arm of the posterior IVS prosthesis did retract unilaterally over the vaginal vault resulting in a fibrous band. Unilateral section of this band has resolved the problem but did not bring back the symptoms of prolapse.

The eight immediate failures to repair a cystocele, diagnosed on the first follow-up after six weeks and a further three after six months are due to a failure of insertion of the prosthesis between the bladder and the vagina at the level of the vaginal vault or at the level of the uterine isthmus as confirmed during repeat surgery. One of the possible explanation is a lack of length of the prosthesis. During the first operation, the prosthesis measured 6 cm gendering an excessive tension when the vaginal vault was hauled towards the sacrum by the posterior IVS. Another hypothesis is that this prosthesis does not treat the "lateral defect." Both explanations have lead, after the experience in the first series of 100 patient, to reconsider the design of the prosthesis. It has been made longer to allow no tension at all and anchoring to the lateral side on the arcus tendineus of the levator ani muscles near the ischial spines in the para rectal fossae.

One complete failure was registered where there has been a reappearance of a cystocele and uterine prolapse at the visit of one year. At the start, there had been a reappearance of the anterior part. The cystocele had pulled on the isthmic region and had gendered the relaxation of the posterior IVS. The patient was treated with a bilateral spinofixation and by bringing the posterior IVS back under tension. It has been noted that in this case the tension on the initial prostheses had been exaggerated. The anterior prosthesis has been reattached laterally to the arcus tendineus musculus levator ani on both sides.

It is still too early to discuss eventual failures considering the short follow-up. The maximal follow-up is of two years. In the small series under scrutiny, however, there have not been other problems.

Discussing the Technique

Posterior IVS is an Australian technique ideated by Petros (7) and in a series published by Farnsworth (8). In our series, however, the original technique has been altered. In our series the rectum has been completely liberated to the lateral side wall as to open the para rectal fossae and this for three reasons. First to protect the rectum during the passage of the "tunneler" without having a finger in the lumen of the rectum. This last maneuver is incompatible with the asepsis needed during the use of prostheses. Second to find the anatomical landmarks (ischial spine, sacro spinal ligament) that allows to place the IVS prosthesis and to haul the vaginal vault into the right direction versus S3. Finally, to allow the placement of a prosthesis between the rectum and the vagina to reinforce the fascia as to avoid the classical suturing together of the musculi levatores ani. This latter technique reduces the diameter of the vagina and cause frequent complaints of dysparoenia. The incision for the colpography has also been modified. A saggital medial incision is used. This incision allows for easy access to the para rectal fossae and because this incision plane is perpendicular to the plane of the posterior IVS there is less erosion of this prosthesis. With this modified technique we did not observe erosions in this series.

The authors believe that the reduced percentage of erosions is due to the tension-free placement and positioning of the prosthesis deep between the fascia (fascia left as an integral part of the vaginal mucosa) and the organ. This technique respects the vascularization of the vaginal epithelium decreasing the risk of necrosis uncovering parts of the prosthesis. The low incidence of infections is entirely due to the extreme measures to maintain an absolute sterility during the placement of the prosthesis; a second disinfection of the perineal area, the covering of the anal sphincter with a transparent adhesive film, systematic antibiotic prophylaxis, changing of gloves after every single manipulation of the prostheses, no rectal examination as long as not all incisions are closed, last minute opening of the packs containing the polypropylene mesh. The authors wish to recommend this way taking care of sterility as infection of the prosthesis nearly always occurs during the operation brought into the field by the surgeon.

CONCLUSION

It is the author's opinion that posterior IVS greatly simplifies the treatment of vaginal vault prolapse, uterine descent and enterocele. The technique could become an interesting alternative for the spinofixation. This point has been evaluated in a prospective randomized trial. Combined with the placement of prosthesis between the vagina and the bladder and one between the rectum and the vagina, the technique can be called the triple perineal operation. This technique offers a global solution to the problem of combined descent comparable to the promonto-fixation. The same prostheses are placed in the same planes. The reduction in theater time and the short learning curve will allow this technique to become a strong concurrent for the classical technique that has been performed by laparotomy or by laparoscopy for over 40 years.

REFERENCES

1. Constantin S, Iosif CS. Abdominal sacral colpopexy using synthetic mesh. Acta Obstet Gynecol Scand 1993; 72:214–7.
2. Cheret A, van Theobald P, Lucas J, Dreyfus M, Herlicoviez M. Faisabilité de la promontofixation par voie coelioscopique. Série prospective de 44 cas. J Gynecol Obstet Bio Reprod 2001; 30:139–43.

3. Cosson M, Bogaert E, Nzarducci F, Querleu D, Crepin G. Promontofixation par coelioscopie:résultats à court terme et complications chez 88 patientes. J Gynecol Obstet Bio Reprod 2000; 29:746–50.
4. Mahedran D, Prasmar S, Smith ARB, Murphy O. Laparoscopic sacrocolpopexy in the management of vaginal vault prolapse. Gynecol Endosc 1996; 5:217–22.
5. Nezhat CH, Nezhat F, Nezhat C. Laparoscopic sacrocolpopexy for vaginal vault prolapse. Obstet Gynecol 1994; 84:885–8.
6. Bum RC, Mattiasson A, Bo K, Brubaker LP, DeLancey JOL, Klarskov P, Shull BL, Smith ARB. The standardization of terminology of female pelvic organ prolapse and pelvic floor dysfunction. Am J Obstet Gynecol 1996; 175:10–7.
7. Petros PE. Vault prolapse II: restoration of dynamic vaginal supports by infracoccygeal sacropexy, an axial day-case vaginal procedure. Int Urogynecol J Pelvic Floor Dysfunct 2001; 12(5):296–303.
8. Farnsworth BN. Posterior intravaginal slingplasty (infracoccygeal sacropexy) for severe posthysterectomy vaginal vault prolapse: a preliminary report on efficacy and safety. Int Urogynecol J Pelvic Floor Dysfunct 2002; 13(1):4–8.

12

Vaginal Vault Prolapse: Sacrofixation

Jacques Donnez, Jean-Paul Squifflet, Pascale Jadoul, and Mireille Smets
Department of Gynecology, Université Catholique de Louvain, Cliniques Universitaires Saint-Luc, Brussels, Belgium

The surgical treatment of vaginal vault prolapse and cervical or uterine prolapse is a major challenge to the surgeon, especially when preservation of sexual function is sought. In patients with surgical contraindications, the placement of a vaginal pessary may offer great relief from symptoms without any surgical risk. But when surgery is possible, it is the preferable mode of therapy.

Genital prolapse can be treated by various techniques, with or without synthetic material (prosthesis), by laparotomy, laparoscopy, or a vaginal approach. In vaginal surgery, hysterectomy is usually associated with the technique, except in case of transposition of the uterosacral ligaments in front of the cervix (Shirodkar technique). Fixation of the vagina to the sacrospinous ligament by the vaginal route has been described (1). Access by laparotomy may be associated with total hysterectomy, subtotal hysterectomy or uterus conservation. A synthetic material is then often used to attach the cervix, the uterus or the vagina to the sacrum or the prevertebral ligament. Alloplastic graft materials such as polytetrafluoroethylene (Teflon®) (2,3), propylene (Marlex®) (2,4–6), polyester fiber (Mersilene®) (2,7–11), Gore Tex® (2,7) or polypropylene (12) have been used by many authors. Homologous materials such as fascia (13–15) or dura mater (16) have also been used and well tolerated, although non-absorbable sutures covered with peritoneum have been reported (17). Since 1993, laparoscopic procedures have been proposed for the management of vaginal, cervical or uterine prolapse (18–21). All of these techniques use synthetic material that attaches the vagina or the cervix to the promonto-sacral space (18,20) or the antero-superior iliac spine (19), according to the technique described by Kapandji (22). Uterine promonto-sacropexy is, at present, the most frequently used technique in young women.

A series of 98 women underwent a simple combined vaginal and laparoscopic procedure with or without uterus conservation, consisting of the sacral fixation of a tightened polypropylene prosthesis (mesh) attached to the posterior part of the cervix or the vaginal vault. This mesh was fixed to the body of either the first sacral vertebra or the fifth lumbar vertebra with the help of a novel tacking device (Origin TackerÔ Fixation Device, Origin Medsystems, Inc., Menlo Park, CA, USA). All the women had a preoperative front and profile lumbosacral junction X-ray to check the promontory. This chapter evaluates the 5-year results in this series of 98 patients.

OPERATIVE TECHNIQUE

Cervical or Uterine Sacrofixation

The patient is placed in the Trendelenburg position. The surgeon is on the left of the patient and holds the laparoscope in his right hand. The assistant is between the legs of the patient. Single-tooth vulsellum forceps are placed on the anterior lip of the cervix and a cannula is inserted into the cervix for uterine mobilization if the cervix is present. A Foley catheter is inserted into the bladder. Three 5-mm suprapubic trocars are introduced: one in the midline and two lateral to the epigastric vessels.

First Step: Exploration

- The abdominal cavity is explored first. The peritoneum, the uterus and the adnexa are inspected; the ureters are traced along the pelvic side wall and the major iliac vessels are carefully located. Adhesiolysis is performed if necessary. A laparoscopic subtotal hysterectomy (LASH) may be performed if indicated (23,24). The uterine corpus should then be removed during the second step (colpotomy).

Second Step: Cervical Fixation of the Mesh by Posterior Colpotomy

- After careful disinfection of the Douglas pouch and the vagina with an iodine solution, a posterior colpotomy is performed using a sagittal vaginal incision over a length of 4 to 5 cm. After the dissection and opening of the posterior peritoneal cul-de-sac, a right-angled retractor is placed on the posterior lip of the vagina. Another vulsellum holds the posterior lip of the cervix to provide exposure. If LASH was performed during the first step, the uterus would have been removed already. A polypropylene mesh is then tightly stitched to the posterior part of the cervix with two non-absorbable stitches (Nylon 0, Ethicon, Somerville, USA) (due to the risk of vaginal erosion, only absorbable sutures are presently used). The mesh is placed in the abdominal cavity. Two round circumferential sutures are then placed high on the peritoneum in order to carry out a culdoplasty to treat associated enterocele. The highest suture brings together the uterosacral ligaments to the midline to prevent any future occurrence. The culdotomy is then closed using an interrupted or running suture.

Third Step: Laparoscopic Dissection of the Presacral Tissue

- The patient, still in the Trendelenburg position, is placed in slightly left lateral decubitus. After careful coagulation of the peritoneum, an opening is made with scissors from the lumbosacral joint towards the cervix. The prevertebral space is opened. The presacral peritoneum is grasped with two atraumatic forceps on the right lateral side of the rectum. The right ureter is situated 1 to 2 cm from the presacral peritoneal incision and is systematically checked over the length of this incision. The sigmoid is pushed laterally and careful dissection and hemostasis of the presacral tissue provides exposure of the anterior common vertebral ligament. Coagulation and section of the medial sacral artery and vein are sometimes necessary. The most prominent point of the space is the lumbosacral joint. The mesh must be fixed either to the anterior wall of the corpus of the first sacral vertebra or to that of the fifth lumbar vertebra.

Fourth Step: Sacral Fixation of the Polypropylene Mesh

- Two grasping forceps hold the edges of the parietal posterior peritoneum to give access to the anterior wall of the first sacral vertebra. The Origin TackerÔ is introduced through the medial suprapubic trocar. This tacking device utilizes a helical coil of 3.9 mm in diameter to achieve secure fixation to the vertebra. Forceps grasp the mesh, which is then tightened until the cervix or the uterus recovers its anatomical position. The tip of the TackerÔ is placed on the mesh, in front of the anterior wall of the first sacral vertebra, and several tacks are inserted through the mesh into the periosteum of the vertebra and the common vertebral ligament. Excess mesh is cut away and removed (Figs. 1 and 2).

Fifth Step: Reperitonealization

- Both folds of the peritoneum are sutured with a resorbable material or stapled with endoscopic staples. Careful washing of the peritoneal cavity is then performed and an antiseptic solution of Rifocine (Rifamycin, Merrel Dow, Kansas City, USA) is instilled into the pelvis. Finally, a catheter is placed into the pouch of Douglas through one of the suprapubic trocars. It is clamped for 2 to 4 h and removed the day after surgery.

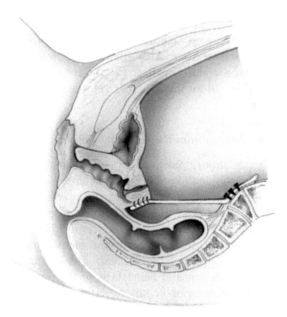

Figure 1   Sacral fixation of the polypropylene mesh. A polypropylene mesh is fixed vaginally to the cervix or the vaginal vault.

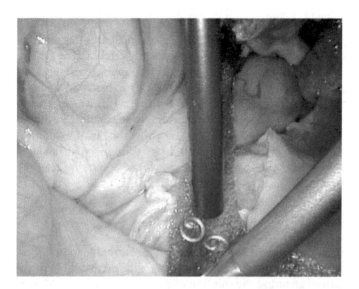

Figure 2   The tip of the Tacker System (Origin, Autosuture) is placed on the mesh in front of the anterior wall of the first sacral vertebra, and several tacks are inserted through the mesh into the periosteum of the vertebra.

Vaginal Vault Sacrofixation

Fixation of the mesh to the vagina can be done either vaginally or laparoscopically using the tacking technique, but the vaginal route is preferred because it allows quick repair of enterocele.

Using the vaginal route, the vagina is opened along its posterior wall with a 4 to 5 cm-long incision perpendicular to the vaginal vault. Dissection is performed to enter the abdominal cavity. The enterocele is then dissected and the excess peritoneum cut away.

The polypropylene mesh is fixed to the vaginal vault through the vaginal incision with two or three non-absorbable stitches. The mesh is introduced into the peritoneal cavity. The peritoneum is then closed with two high continuous round circumferential sutures to close the pouch of Douglas (Douglasorrhaphy). The vagina is finally closed.

It is important to note that none of our patients underwent a concomitant Burch procedure.

After surgery, a pessary is placed, which is removed 1 month later during the postoperative check-up. On postoperative day 3, a radiography of the sacrum is obtained to confirm the correct position of the coils.

COMPLICATIONS

We did not observe any intraoperative complications. No bleeding occurred during the procedure among the 98 patients in this study. There was one immediate postoperative complication (Table 1). One patient complained of difficulty moving her left foot immediately after leaving the operating room. It was associated with severe pain in the left buttock and in the upper part of the left thigh. An electromyography concluded that the fifth left lumbar neural root or one of the first left sacro-neural roots was affected. A radiography of the sacrum showed that one coil was too laterally placed on the left, near the neural root. After confirmation by magnetic resonance imaging (MRI) that one spring had been placed in the foramen intervertebrale of the second sacral root, we decided to perform a laparotomy and the spring was carefully removed. The patient

Table 1 Complications and Recurrence after Laparoscopic Sacrofixation ($n = 98$)

Complications:	
Compression of sciatic nerve (wrong insertion)	$n = 1$
Spondylodiscitis	$n = 2$
Vaginal erosion (only in case of vaginal vault prolapse)	$n = 3$
Recurrence:	
Defective application to the cervix	$n = 2$
Enterocele after vaginal vault prolapse without enterocele repair	$n = 1$

made a rapid recovery and, six months after surgery, had only a slight mobility defect of her left foot.

Postoperative discomfort was similar to that observed after any straightforward laparoscopy. Bowel function resumed within 24 hr and the patients were able to leave hospital on average on day 2 to 4 postoperatively. Sexual intercourse was allowed three weeks after surgery. Patients were reviewed every six months. The follow-up in this series is now longer than five years. Two patients experienced spondylodiscitis, nine months and fifteen days postoperatively. The first one underwent laparotomy with disc resection and bone transplantation. The second was treated by laparoscopy, during which the mesh and coils were removed.

We observed three cases of recurrence. The first case was observed 8 months after surgery. The patient underwent another laparoscopy, which showed that the mesh was well fixed to the sacrum but detached from the cervix. The mesh was separated from the covering peritoneum and then fixed to the cervix with the help of two non-absorbable sutures. The second case of recurrence was due to incomplete surgery. Indeed, this patient, who had undergone fixation of the vaginal vault, developed a severe enterocele several months later. She underwent surgery a second time and laparoscopy showed that the vaginal vault was well fixed to the mesh, but an enterocele had developed below the point of fixation of the mesh to the vagina. Vaginal surgery of the enterocele was easily carried out. The third case of recurrence was observed after three years, probably due to great exertion on the part of the patient.

COMMENTS

The goal of pelvic reconstruction is to restore normal anatomy, maintain or restore normal bladder and bowel function, and provide a vagina of normal length to ensure pain-free coitus (25). A well-supported vagina lies on the rectum and levator plate with its axis directed towards the hollow of the sacrum and its apex at or above the ischial spines. It is suspended from the sacrum by the paracolpium. Vaginography (26) and contemporary MRI demonstrate this anatomical fact. Vaginal eversion and uterine prolapse are a result of disruption of the upper paracolpium, which includes the fibromuscular tissue of the cardinal and uterosacral ligaments (20). Many different corrective procedures use this anatomical principle and anchor the vaginal apex or the cervix to the available supporting tissue at this level, including the sacrospinous ligaments, iliococcygeus or coccygeus fascia, uterosacral ligaments, or sacrum.

Many authors have advocated a purely vaginal approach for this condition. The main problem is that in case of severe attenuation of both uterosacral ligaments, which is frequent in vaginal vault prolapse, vaginal repair of cystocele and rectocele often fails (27). The technique, first proposed by Amreich (28) and later modified by Richter and Albrich, involves fixation of the vaginal vault to the sacrospinous ligament (1).

One of the disadvantages of sacrospinous ligament fixation is the marked vaginal retroversion that results from this type of fixation; this may predispose the patient to recurrent support defects in the anterior vagina, resulting in cystocele, urethral hypermobility, or both (29,30). Holley et al. (30) reported a 92% incidence of cystocele (76% first-degree and 24% second-degree) in 36 women who underwent sacrospinous ligament fixation or repair of associated pelvic support defects during a mean follow-up period of 42 months. The majority of cases were asymptomatic, however, and only a small number required a subsequent surgical procedure (5.5%). A second disadvantage of sacrospinous ligament fixation is the possible neuropathy produced by the vaginal dissection (31). Such neuropathy may have an effect on subsequent muscle strength and integrity of muscular tissue support. It can also cause lower urinary tract dysfunction and explain the higher incidence of incontinence after sacrospinous ligament fixation than after sacrofixation (32).

In a prospective study comparing the vaginal versus the abdominal approach, Benson et al. (32) demonstrated that the abdominal approach is more effective at treating uterovaginal prolapse, with the probability for an optimal surgical outcome twice as great as with the vaginal approach.

Among the transabdominal approaches described so far, the most frequently published is fixation of the vaginal vault to the midsacrum or sacral promontory using an artificial material. Sacral colpopexy has a high success rate (85% to 99%) in vault prolapse repair and does not shorten the vagina (5,6,8,33–35).

Laparoscopic approaches to sacrofixation (12,20,36) have been described, and may be compared to the more traditional laparotomy approaches (Table 2). The advantage of sacrofixation is that it ensures vaginal length with a larger caliber, normal horizontal vaginal axis and a more anatomical repair (37). Sacral colpopexy is performed to correct severe vaginal vault eversion by replacing the upper paracolpium with synthetic mesh, which results in a stronger fixation than a simple culdoplasty (20). According to Ameline and Huguier (38), the only truly physiological suspension involves placement of suture material into the ligamentous and periosteal fibrous connective tissue in the midline of the anterior sacrum. Although sacral segments 3 and 4 are anatomically ideal, control of the tip of the needle deep in the hollow of the sacrum is difficult and laceration of presacral veins is an ever-present risk, leading to life-threatening hemorrhage, which is extremely difficult to control (39). Fixation to the first vertebra (beyond the sacrolumbar joint) or the lower part of the fifth lumbar vertebra gives back the genital tube its triple angulation: posteroascending vaginal obliquity, anteflexion of the cervix over the uterine corpus and anteversion. It thus correctly restores the anatomy.

Table 2 Long-Term Results of the Surgical Approach

Reference	No. of patients	Follow-up (years)	Success rate (%)
Lefranc and Blondon (45)	316	10	>90
Ocelli et al. (46)	271	1–11	97.7
Deval et al. (47)	232	1–12	91.1
Lecuru et al. (48)	203	1-7	86.7
Snyder et al. (7)	147	5	93
Valattis and Stanton (49)	41	10	88
Donnez et al. (50)	98	5	96
von Theobald and Chéret (51)	100	4	96

In one of our previous series of cases where sacrofixation was performed by laparotomy or laparoscopy (12) using MackarÔ staples, severe cystoceles were not observed (except in two cases), even after long-term follow-up. This is probably due to the more anatomical reconstruction. Like Hoff (40), we believe that, in the great majority of cases, anterior colporrhaphy with sacrofixation is not needed to treat an associated cystocele. Nevertheless, we believe that posterior colporrhaphy can be helpful to treat even a huge rectocele. We performed posterior colporrhaphy only in cases where the rectocele was so large that simple fixation of the cervix or vagina would not allow sufficient reduction.

Like Smith (6), we believe that fixation of the prosthesis to the bone is stronger than suturing it to the sacrospinous ligament. In one of our previous series of 20 patients treated between 1985 and 1995, we anchored the prosthesis to the bone using MackarÔ staples by laparotomy or laparoscopy. The long-term results were excellent and no recurrence was noted (12). The tacking technique described here allows fixation of the mesh to the vertebra with the same reliability. It is less invasive since only the periosteum is penetrated; this reduces the risk of bone infection. It avoids difficulties associated with placement of prevertebral sutures. The most common complications of sacropexy are intraoperative bleeding and postoperative fever. With this approach, spondylodiscitis and bleeding due to presacral vessel lesions are rarely observed (39,41,42). The mesh should be reperitonealized to prevent bowel adhesions (43,44). Undue tension must be avoided to prevent pain (5).

We observed prolapse recurrence in three of the 98 patients who underwent sacrofixation (3.4%). The first occurred in a patient in whom the mesh had been fixed to the cervix using coil. It was the cervical fixation of the mesh that had given way, while the sacral fixation remained intact. The consistency of the cervix does not favor fixation of the mesh using tacking springs and requires the use of non-absorbable sutures. We prefer to do this by posterior colpotomy.

This allows the surgeon to perform a Douglasorrhaphy, shorten the uterosacral ligaments and treat the enterocele, if present, at the same time. The second case of recurrence also involved an enterocele. It was explained by the fact that simple fixation of the mesh to the vagina is not sufficient because it could promote, as in this case, the development of a more severe enterocele by "sliding" under the site of fixation. For this reason, Douglasorrhaphy and enterocele repair must be systematically carried out in case of vaginal vault repair. The third case was a prolapse recurrence, necessitating a second procedure.

Sacrofixation, in contrast to sacrospinous ligament fixation, is a more anatomical repair. It does not favor development of a secondary cystocele, it does not cause vaginal shortening and, provided that prevertebral dissection is well performed and particular care is taken to insert the springs into the central part of the body of the vertebra, it is without risk for the nerves. Difficulties can be encountered in overweight women who have a deep layer of adipose tissue between the prevertebral peritoneum and the vertebral bone itself.

CONCLUSION

A combined vaginal and laparoscopic approach is preferable for the surgical treatment of uterine or vaginal vault prolapse. Fixation of the mesh by posterior colpotomy has several advantages. First, it allows easy use of strong sutures. Second, additional procedures can be performed to treat or prevent enterocele. Third, this approach is associated with a shorter operative time compared to a purely laparoscopic approach.

Laparoscopic fixation of the mesh to the sacrum with the help of springs (Origin TackerÔ System) also has several advantages. It avoids the risk of presacral vein laceration that may be caused by the use of a needle. It provides easy and quick fixation of the mesh to the fifth lumbar vertebra or the first sacral vertebra. Finally, it gives an extremely good quality fixation.

REFERENCES

1. Richter K, Albrich W. Long-term results following fixation of the vagina on the sacrospinal ligament by the vaginal route (vaginal fixation sacrospinalis vaginalis). Am J Obstet Gynecol 1981; 141:811.
2. Virtanen H, Hirvonen T, Mäkinen J, Kiilholna P. Outcome of thirty patients who underwent repair of posthysterectomy prolapse of the vaginal vault with abdominal sacral colpopexy. J Am Coll Surg 1994; 178:283.
3. Birnboum SJ. Rational therapy for the prolapsed vagina. Am J Obstet Gynecol 1973; 115:411.
4. Grundsell H, Lorsson G. Operative management of vaginal vault prolapse following hysterectomy. Br J Obstet Gynecol 1984; 91:808.

5. Drutz HP, Cha LS. Massive genital and vaginal vault prolapse treated by abdominal vaginal sacropexy with the use of Marlex Mesh. Review of the literature. Am J Obstet Gynecol 1987; 156:387.

6. Smith MR. Colposacropexy: an alternative technique. Am J Obstet Gynecol 1997; 176:1374–5.

7. Snyder TE, Krantz KE, Litt D. Abdominal retroperitoneal sacral colpopexy for the correction of vaginal prolapse. Obstet Gynecol 1991; 77:944.

8. Addison WA, Timmons MC, Wall LL MD, Livengood CH. Failed abdominal sacral colpopexy: observations and recommendations. Obstet Gynecol 1989; 74: 480–2.

9. Rust JA, Botte JM, Howlett RJ. Prolapse of the vaginal vault. Improved techniques for the management of the abdominal approach or vaginal approach. Am J Obstet Gynecol 1976; 125:768.

10. Creighton SM, Stanton SL. The surgical management of vaginal vault prolapse. Br J Obstet Gynecol 1991; 98:1150.

11. Timmons MC, Addison WA, Addison SB, Cavenar MG. Abdominal sacral colpopexy in 163 women with posthysterectomy vaginal vault prolapse and enterocele. J Reprod Med 1992; 37:323.

12. Smets M, Donnez J. Mackar staple fixation for uterus prolapse. Gynecol Endoscopy 1995; 4(1):18.

13. Maloney JC, Dunton CJ, Smith K. Repair of vaginal vault prolapse with abdominal sacropexy. J Reprod Med 1990; 35:6.

14. Hendee AE, Berry CM. Abdominal sacropexy for vaginal vault prolapse. Clin Obstet Gynecol 1981; 24:1217.

15. Kaupilla O, Punnonen R, Teisala K. Operative technique for the repair of posthysterectomy vaginal prolapse. Ann Chir Gynecol 1986; 75:242.

16. Lansman HH. Posthysterectomy vault prolapse: sacral colpopexy with dura mater graft. Obstet Gynecol 1984; 63:577.

17. Grünberger W, Grünberger V, Wierani F. Pelvic promontory fixation of the vaginal vault in sixty-two patients with prolapse after hysterectomy. J Am Coll Surg 1994; 178:69.

18. Querleu D, Parmentier D, Debodinance P. Premiers essais de coeliochirurgie dans le traitement du prolapsus génital et de l'incontinence urinaire d'effort. In Blanc B, Boubli L, Baudrant E, d'Ercale C (eds). Les troubles de la statique pelvienne. Paris: Arnette Editions; 1993, p. 155.

19. Cornier E, Madelenat P. Hystéropexie selon M. Kapandji: technique percoelioscopique et résultats préliminaires. J Gynecol Obstet Biol Reprod 1994; 23:378.

20. Ross JW. Techniques of laparoscopic repair of total vault eversion after hysterectomy. J Am Assoc Gynecol Laparoscopists 1997; 4:173–83.

21. Godin PA, Nisolle M, Smets M, Squifflet J, Donnez J. Combined vaginal and laparoscopic sacrofixation for genital prolapse using a tacking technique: a series of 45 cases. Gynaecol Endoscopy 1999; 8:277–85.

22. Kapandji M. Cure des prolapsus uro-génitaux par colpo-isthmo-cystopexie par bandelettes transversales et la Douglassoraphie ligamento-péritonéale étagée et croisée. Ann Chir 1967; 21:32.

23. Donnez J, Nisolle M. LASH: laparoscopic supracervical (subtotal) hysterectomy. J Gynecol Surg 1993; 9:91–4.
24. Donnez J, Nisolle M, Smets M, Polet R, Bassil S. Laparoscopic supracervical (subtotal) hysterectomy. A first series of 500 cases. Gynaecol Endosc 1997; 6: 73–6.
25. Shull BL, Capen CV, Riggs MW, et al. Preoperative and postoperative analysis of site-specific pelvic support defects in 81 women treated with sacrospinous ligament suspension and pelvic reconstruction. Am J Obstet Gynecol 1992; 166: 1764–71.
26. Nichols DH, Milloy AS, Randall CL. Significance of restoration of normal vaginal depth and axis. Obstet Gynecol 1970; 36:251–5.
27. Symmonds RE, Williams TJ, Lee RA, Webb MJ. Posthysterectomy enterocele and vaginal vault prolapse. Am J Obstet Gynecol 1981; 140:852.
28. Amreich J. Actrologie und Operation des Schidenstrumpf-Prolapses. Wien Klin Wodenschr 1951; 63:74.
29. Cruikshank S, Cox D. Sacrospinous ligament fixation at the time of transvaginal hysterectomy. Am J Obstet Gynecol 1990; 162:1611–9.
30. Holley RL, Varner RE, Gleason BP, et al. Recurrent pelvic support defects after sacrospinous ligament fixation for vaginal vault prolapse. J Am Coll Surg 1995; 180:444–80.
31. Benson JT, McClellan E. The effect of vaginal dissection on the pubertal nerve. Obstet Gynecol 1993; 82:387–9.
32. Benson JT, Lucente V, McClellan E. Vaginal versus abdominal reconstructive surgery for the treatment of pelvic support defects: a prospective randomized study with long-term outcome evaluation. Am J Obstet Gynecol 1996; 175: 1418–22.
33. Arthure HG, Savage D. Uterine prolapse and prolapse of the vagina treated by sacropexy. J Obstet Gynaecol Br Commonw 1957; 64:355–60.
34. Creighton S, Stanton S. The surgical management of vaginal prolapse. Br J Obstet Gynaecol 1991; 98:1150–4.
35. Grunberger W, Grunberger V, Wierrrani F. Pelvic promontory fixation of the vaginal vault in sixty-two patients with prolapse after hysterectomy. J Am Coll Surg 1994; 178:69–72.
36. Nezhat CH, Nezhat F, Nezhat C. Laparoscopic sacral colpopexy for vaginal vault prolapse. Obstet Gynecol 1994; 84:885–8.
37. Vitanen H, Hirvonen T, Makinen J, et al. Outcome of thirty patients who underwent repair of posthysterectomy prolapse of the vaginal vault with abdominal sacral colpopexy. J Am Coll Surg 1994; 178:283–7.
38. Ameline A, Huguier J. La suspension postérieure aux disques lombo-sacrés: technique de remplacement des ligaments utéro-sacrés par voie abdominale. J Gynecol Obstet Biol Reprod 1957; 56:94.
39. Sutton JP, Addison WA, Livengood CH, Hammond CB. Life-threatening hemorrhage complicating sacral colpopexy. Am J Obstet Gynecol 1981; 140:836.
40. Hoff S, Manelfe A, Portet R, Girot C. Promontofixation ou suspension par bandelettes transversables? Etude comparée de ces deux techniques dans le traitement des prolapsus génitaux. Ann Chir 1984; 38:363.

41. Baker KR, Beresford JM, Campbell C. Colposacropexy with Prolene mesh. Obstet Gynecol 1990; 171:51.
42. Addison WA, Livengood CH, Sutton GP, Parker RT. Abdominal sacral colpopexy with Mercilene mesh in the retroperitoneal position in the management of posthysterectomy vaginal vault prolapse and enterocele. Am J Obstet Gynecol 1985; 15:140.
43. Soichet S. Surgical correction of total genital prolapse with retention of sexual function. Obstet Gynecol 1970; 36:69–75.
44. Todd JW. Mesh suspension for vaginal prolapse. Int Surg 1978; 63:91–93.
45. Lefranc JP, Blondon J. Chirurgie des prolapsus génitaux par voie abdominale. J Chir 1983; 120:431–6.
46. Ocelli B, Marducci F, Cosson M, Ego A. La promontofixation par voie abdominale dans la cure des prolapsus génitaux féminins avec ou sans incontinence urinaire. A propos de 271 cas. Ann Chir 1999; 53:367–77.
47. Deval B, Fauconnier A, Repiquet D, Liou Y, Montuclard B. Traitement chirurgical des prolapsus génito-urinaires par voie abdominale. A propos d'une série de 232 cas. Ann Chir 1997; 51:256–65.
48. Lecuru F, Taurelle R, Clouard C, Attal JP. Traitement chirurgical des prolapsus génito-urinaires par voie abdominale. Résultats d'une série continue de 203 interventions. Ann Chir 1994; 48:1013–9.
49. Valattis SR, Stanton SL. A retrospective study of a clinician experience. Br J Obstet Gynecol 1994; 101:518–22.
50. Donnez J, Squifflet J, Smets M, Nisolle M. Laparoscopic sacrofixation. In Donnez J, Nisolle M (eds), An Atlas of Operative Laparoscopy and Hysteroscopy. Carnforth, Lanes, UK, Parthenon Publishers; 2001, pp. 283–93.
51. von Theobald P, Chéret A. Laparoscopic sacrocolpopexy: results of a 100-patient series with 8 years follow-up. Gynecol Surg 2004; 1:31–6.

13

Vaginal Vault Prolapse: Lateral Fixation

Jean Bernard Dubuisson, Sandrine Jacob, and Jean-Marie Wenger
Department of Obstetrics and Gynecology, Hôpitaux Universitaires de Genève, Geneva, Switzerland

Victor Gomel
Department of Obstetrics and Gynecology, Faculty of Medicine, University of British Columbia and Women's Hospital and Health Center, Vancouver, British Columbia, Canada

INTRODUCTION

Over the past 40 years, numerous operative techniques have been reported for the treatment of genital prolapse. The goal of these various techniques is to suspend the vaginal vault, the uterus, the bladder and the rectum correctly, and to repair the pelvic floor. Until recently these procedures were performed by the vaginal route or by laparotomy. Progress in operative laparoscopy makes it possible to treat genital prolapse by laparoscopic access. The laparoscopic procedure employed has been sacrocolpopexy using a technique similar to that performed by laparotomy (1–4). The anatomical and functional results obtained with this procedure are excellent. The laparoscopic sacrocolpopexy is considered as "gold standard" for the surgical treatment of genital prolapse by abdominal route.

The purpose of this chapter is to report our experience with a new laparoscopic technique to treat genital prolapse. Details of the technique of laparoscopic lateral suspension were published in 1998 (5). This technique was inspired from an open abdominal procedure described by Kapandji (6). In the technique published in 1998, lateral colpo-uterine suspension was achieved using two meshes. After the evaluation of the results of this group of patients the technique was modified by using only a single mesh placed as a transversal hammock and sutured at its mid-portion, inferiorly to the pubocervical fascia and pericervical ring; and each end of the mesh attached superiorly to the aponeurosis of the external oblique, on each side. It was found that the second mesh that used to be fixed posteriorly to the rectovaginal septum and the torus uterinum offered no benefits and increased the risk of mesh erosion. This second mesh is no longer used. Instead, a posterior colporrhaphy is performed by laparoscopic access and the uterosacral ligaments are reattached to the apex of the vaginal vault. This new technique is simpler, avoids the risk of vaginal erosion due to the mesh and offers excellent results. Further, it enables complete treatment of genital prolapse by laparoscopic access without use of the promontory and need for extensive peritonealization.

OPERATIVE TECHNIQUE

Preparation of the Patient

All patients are prescribed preoperative bowel preparation, as follows: low residue diet for five days followed by one dose of Colophos Solution® (Spirig laboratories, Switzerland) by mouth given two days before the operation and an enema given on the day before the operation. General anesthesia with endotracheal intubation is used in all cases.

Laparoscopy

The patient is placed in a lithotomy position with the thighs spread moderately and bent upwards. After appropriate preparation and draping, a Foley catheter is inserted in the bladder, and a uterine manipulator is attached to the cervix (when uterus present) (7) for the adequate exposure of the anterior and posterior vaginal fornices. After the establishment of pneumoperitoneum transumbilically, the laparoscope is introduced, and three ancillary suprapubic ports are used to perform the procedure. Two 5 mm trocars are inserted laterally; 3 to 4 cm above the iliac crests and a 10 to 12 mm trocar is inserted in the midline half-way between the umbilicus and the pubis. The peritoneal cavity is then thoroughly inspected with special attention paid to the pelvis. The uterus is evaluated. The ovaries are also inspected. The extent of the genital descent is evaluated; lateral extension of the cystocele, presence of an enterocele, and quality of the uterosacral ligaments is assessed.

Operative Technique

The procedure includes the following steps all performed by laparoscopy.
   The first step is *the dissection of the endopelvic fascias*. The second assistant stands between the patient's legs and holds a foam swab placed on a long forceps or a long retractor to expose the posterior fornix; this facilitates dissection of the tissues in the lower pelvis.

The posterior vaginal wall and the rectovaginal septum are dissected first from the rectum. The peritoneum is incised in the midline between the uterosacral ligaments and the rectum is cleaved from the vagina and the rectovaginal fascia. The extent of the dissection is dependent on the size of the rectocele, and is continued until it reaches the lower part of the defect (Figs. 1 and 2).

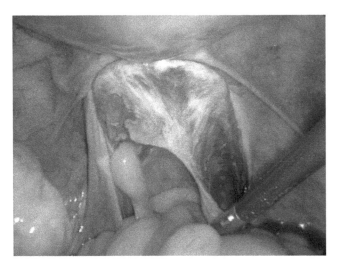

Figure 1   The pouch of Douglas and peritoneal incision between the utero-sacral ligaments.

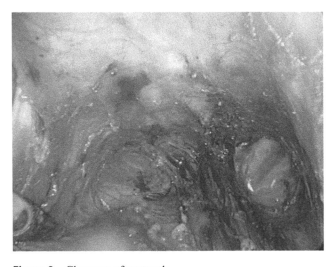

Figure 2   Cleavage of rectocele.

During the dissection, the sacral segments of the uterosacral ligaments are visualized bilaterally; the ureters which are above the ligaments are identified but not dissected.

The anterior vaginal wall and the pubocervical fascia are then freed from the bladder and the dissection carried down to the lower end of the cystocele (Figs. 3 and 4). The lateral extent of the dissection is dependent on the size of the cystocele.

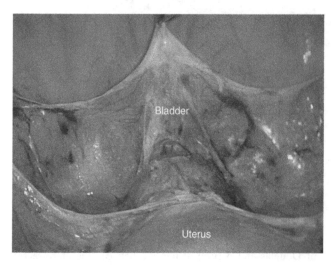

Figure 3   Incision of the anterior pouch.

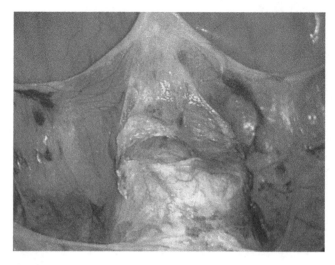

Figure 4   Vesicovaginal cleavage.

The second step is *anterior and posterior colporrhaphy*. Anterior colporrhaphy is carried out first with the plication of the pubocervical fascia This is achieved with interrupted polyester sutures of (Ethibond 0) on a 26 mm curved needle (Fig. 5). At the end of this step the repair is assessed by vaginal examination.

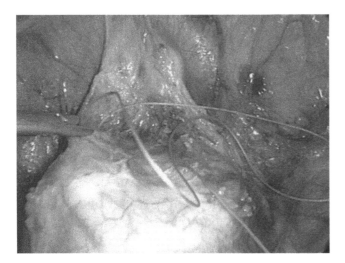

Figure 5   Anterior colporrhaphy.

Posterior colporrhaphy is commenced with the reattachment of the uterosacral ligaments to the torus uterinum. On each side, the sacral segment of the uterosacral ligament is sutured to the rectovaginal fascia, under the rectocele, and to the posterior aspect of the isthmus if the uterus is present, using sutures of Ethibond 0 (Fig. 6). With large rectoceles, we reinforce rectovaginal septum using a rectangular polyester patch. All the fascial sutures are kept extra mucosal to avoid infection and/or erosion. The outcome of this part of the procedure is assessed by vaginal and rectal examination. The reattachment of the uterosacral ligaments usually corrects the uterine prolapse (hysterocele) and reduces the size of the pouch of Douglas which must be partially occluded to prevent a subsequent enterocele.

The third step is the *lateral suspension of the vaginal vault and of the uterus using one mesh, placed as a transversal hammock*. A long strip of polyester mesh of 30 cm long and 3 cm wide with an anterior flap is prepared. The prepared mesh is introduced in the peritoneal cavity through the midline suprapubic trocar. The middle part of this strip is fixed to the anterior and lateral surfaces of the uterine isthmus and to the pubocervical fascia

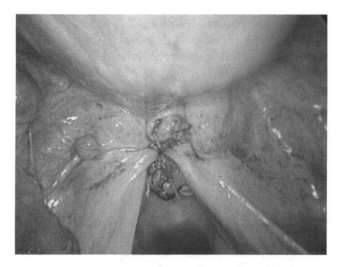

Figure 6 Approximation of the uterosacral ligaments and posterior colograpy completed.

with two separate polyester sutures (Ethibond 0), or to the vaginal vault in a patient who had a prior total hysterectomy (Fig. 7).

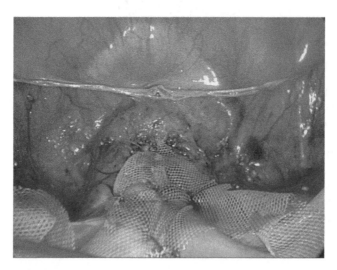

Figure 7 Fixation of the middle part of the mesh to the anterior isthmus and pubocervical fascia.

The transversal hammock is placed laterally by *the fixation of the mesh to the lateral abdominal wall, above the iliac crests*. This requires the creation of the two lateral retroperitoneal tunnels, one on each side. A small cutaneous incision is made 2 cm above and 4 cm lateral to the anterior superior iliac spine. The skin and aponeurosis of the external oblique muscle are incised for about 0.5 cm (Fig. 8). Through theis incision a laparoscopic atraumatic forceps is introduced (Fig. 9) and advanced downwards subperitonealy

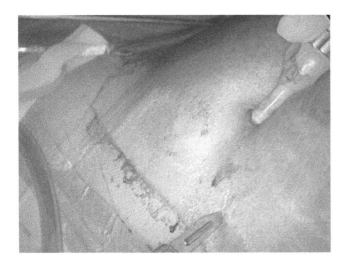

Figure 8 Skin incision on the left lower quadrant to create a retro peritoneal tunnel for the passage of the mesh.

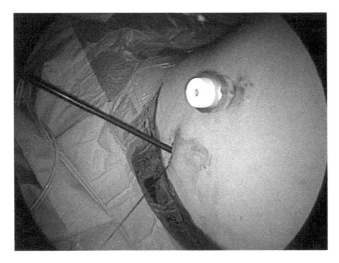

Figure 9 Introduction of a laparoscopic grasping forceps through the incision.

passing under the ipsilateral round ligament and exiting through the supravesical peritoneal incision (Fig. 10). This tunnelling procedure is performed easily under visual control. The distal end of the mesh is grasped by the laparoscopic atraumatic forceps and pulled out of the cutaneous incision above the iliac crest (Fig. 11). The same procedure is repeated on the

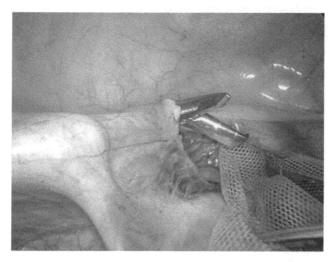

Figure 10   Retroperitoneal tunnelization under the round ligament, on the left side.

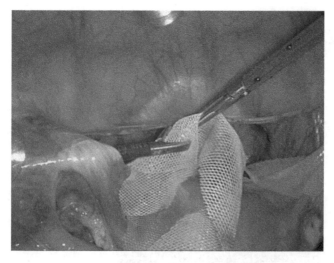

Figure 11   The forceps grasp the distal portion of the mesh, which is pulled out through the retroperitoneal tunnel and skin incision.

opposite side (Figs. 12, 13, and 14). The tension of the hammock is adjusted so that the vaginal vault is suspended at the desired level. Temporary deflation of the pneumoperitoneum permits proper performance of this important step of the procedure. The protruding ends of the meshes are fixed bilaterally to the aponeurosis of the external oblique muscles, using separate interrupted 0 Vicryl sutures.

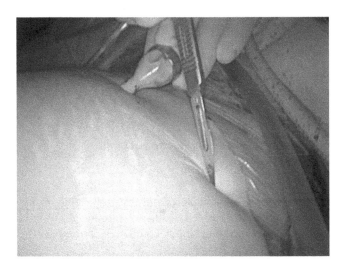

Figure 12 Skin incision on the right lower quadrant.

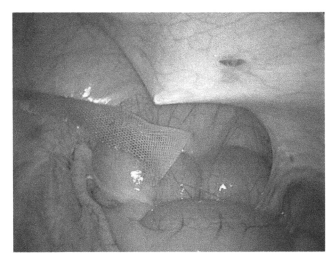

Figure 13 Creation of the retroperitoneal tunnel on the right side.

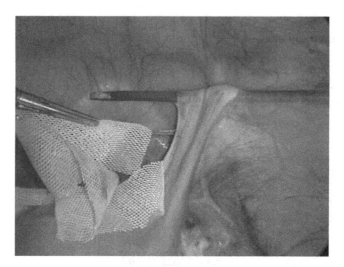

Figure 14   Creation of the retroperitoneal tunnel on the right side.

The fourth step is the *re-peritonealization of the vesico-uterine fornix* (Fig. 15). Reperitonealization is performed using a running 2-0 Vicryl suture. This step is designed to have the mesh completely buried in the retroperitoneal space (Fig. 16).

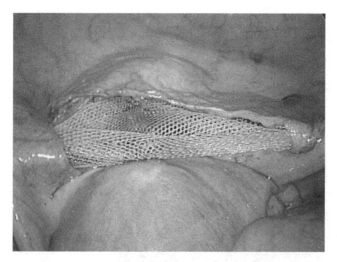

Figure 15   Vesico cervical aspect of the pelvis with central portion of the mesh fixed to the cervix, after tension and before reperitonealization.

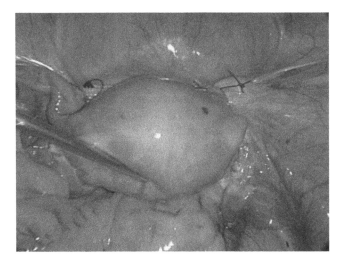

Figure 16 Final aspect of the procedure, after peritonealization.

Associated Procedures

In the presence of benign uterine pathology associated with the genital pro-lapse, a laparoscopic hysterectomy may be indicated. This is discussed pre-operatively with the patient. In such a case, if the cervix is normal we prefer to perform a subtotal hysterectomy as opposed to a total hysterectomy. Available evidence suggests that total hysterectomy increases the risk of infection and secondary erosion of the mesh at the level of the vaginal vault.

In the presence of urinary stress incontinence (USI) or when an important transmission defect is observed during the urodynamic test, a laparoscopic Burch procedure is carried out during the same operation. After dissection of the Retzius' space, the colposuspension is achieved with two sutures of polyester (Ethibon O) placed on each side in the Cooper ligament and in the anterior vaginal wall, opposite the urethro-vesical junction. In the presence of perineal muscles defects a posterior colpoper-ineorrhaphy with rectovaginal fascia repair, using the vaginal approach. Perioperative antibiotic therapy is systematically prescribed. The patient is allowed to leave the hospital as soon as micturition and passage of gas have resumed normally.

PATIENTS, MATERIALS, AND METHODS

A prospective longitudinal case study (unpublished data) was performed between January 1, 2003 and June 30, 2006, 42 patients underwent laparoscopic surgical treatment for genital prolapse using the technique described above in the Department of Obstetrics and Gynecology of the

University Hospitals of Geneva (9). All 133 patients had failed to respond to pelvic floor exercises. Attention was paid to the following parameters: (*i*) Patient characteristics: age, parity, menopausal status, previous history of surgery for USI and genital prolapse. (*ii*) Functional symptoms: degree of prolapse; any other surgical procedures associated with the laparoscopic treatment for prolapse. Urodynamic assessment was performed as necessary. (*iii*) Peri and postoperative complications, duration of the operation, and hospitalization were noted. (*iv*) The efficiency of the operation was assessed from both the anatomical and the functional points of view. The patients came for postoperative consultation at 1, 3, and 6 months and thereafter every year if possible.

Since the procedure was a modification of an existing procedure that had been performed for many years (6), albeit by laparotomy, institutional committee approval was not sought. However, the patients were thoroughly counselled regarding the new technique and possible complications that could ensue.

The mean age of patients was 55.6 ± 54 years (range 34–81); the BMI was 26.75 ± 4.54 (18–37), and the mean parity 2.19 ± 1.18 (range 0–9). Eighty-five patients (63.9%) were menopausal. The genital prolapse characteristics were based on the Pelvic Organ Prolapse Quantification Classification (9). A cystocele Stage 2 or more was noted in 91.7%, a uterine prolapse of stage 2 or more in 66.1%, and a rectocele stage 2 or more in 55.6% of the cases (Table 1).

Table 1 Pre- and Postoperative Components of Genital Prolapse ($n = 133$)

Genital prolapse		Preoperative		Postoperative	
		n	%	*n*	%
Anterior vaginal wall	Stage 0	8	6, 2	122	91.7
	1	3	2, 22	6	4, 5
	2	70	52, 7	4	3
	3	51	38, 3	1	0, 8
	4	1	0, 8	0	0, 8
Hysterocele	Stage 0	10	7, 6	124	93, 2
	1	35	26, 3	5	3, 8
	2	67	50, 4	3	2, 2
	3	18	13, 5	1	0, 8
	4	3	2, 2	0	0, 8
Posterior vaginal wall	Stage 0	17	12, 8	120	90, 2
	1	42	31, 6	9	6, 8
	2	60	45, 1	4	3
	3	14	10, 5	0	0, 8
	4	0	0	0	0, 8

RESULTS

All 42 patients had an anterior and posterior colporrhaphy, a reattachment of the uterosacral ligaments to the apex or the vaginal vault, and a lateral suspension using a single mesh as described. The following surgical procedures were associated with the operation: subtotal hysterectomy ($n = 7$, 16.6%), laparoscopic Burch colposuspension ($n = 22$, 52.38%). The operating time was 191.95 ± 46.43 (120–360) minutes. No patient required blood transfusion. One perioperative complication occurred (2.38%): a bladder injury was observed during the dissection of the pubocervical fascia; the defect was immediately sutured laparoscopicaly with good outcome. Two postoperative complications (4.76%) were noted: one patient required a postoperative blood transfusion subsequent to a hematoma of the Retzius space, after a Burch procedure, which resolved spontaneously; another patient suffered a lateral abdominal wall neuralgia treated by removal of the suture of the mesh to the aponeurosis of the external oblique muscle, under local anesthesia.

The follow up period was 3.02 ± 2.72 (1–12 months). From the functional point of view, two patients experienced de novo USI in the first postoperative week and one had the sensation of uterine descent at 6 months. Thirty-nine patients were satisfied (92.85%). From the anatomical point of view the results were excellent ($n = 41$, 97.6%). In one case a recurrent hysterocele (stage 2) was noted.

Improvements and innovation in laparoscopic instrumentation combined with the increasing experience of the surgeons have permitted performance of more complex operations by laparoscopic access. Several authors, including ourselves, have reported on laparoscopic surgical treatment of genital prolapse (9–12). Laparoscopic sacral colpopexy is now considered the reference technique to treat genital prolapse. This is an approach that is specially used in younger women because of the excellent long-term results, and in women who are sexually active, because of the markedly reduced risk of dyspareunia, due to the absence of vaginal scars (13).

This laparoscopic procedure that combines lateral suspension using a mesh together with anterior and posterior colporrhaphy conforms to the pelvic anatomy and addresses the requirements for correction of pelvic support defects. This technique also conforms to the principles of pelvic support described by De Lancey (14). Level 1 axe defects are corrected with this technique by suspension of the vagina and the cervical ring with a mesh, and the reattachment of the uterosacral ligaments to the rectovaginal fascia and the torus uterinum. Level 2 axe defects are also corrected with the technique described herein. Reconstruction of the anterior support is achieved with plication of the pubocervical fascia (anterior colporrhaphy), and the posterior support by plication of the rectovaginal septum (posterior colporrhaphy).

In laparoscopic treatment of genital prolapse, the use of lateral suspension versus sacral fixation may be a matter of debate. With lateral suspension the risk of complications is very low (2.38%). No vascular complications have been reported. Nezhat et al. (2) treated 15 patients by laparoscopic sacrocolpopexy. One of these had a serious complication that required conversion to laparotomy. In another, a vascular injury occurred during dissection of the promontory. The risk of injury to the vessels located close to the promontory is not specific to the laparoscopic approach. In fact this complication has been reported with a frequency of 1.6% to 4% during sacrocolpopexy via laparotomy (15–17). Although no severe infectious complication has been reported to date during laparoscopic sacrocolpopexy, there is a theoretical risk of sacral osteitis. One investigator has reported such a complication after sacrocolpopexy by laparotomy (18). It is largely because of the markedly reduced risk of these two complications that we consider laparoscopic lateral suspension a preferable alternative for the treatment of genital prolapse. The satisfactory outcomes associated with this approach have been corroborated in several publications (19–21).

Mesh erosion is a complication that is not infrequently observed (15). We did have such complications with our earlier technique (9), but with our current approach we did not have complications related to the mesh. The technique of lateral suspension has been criticized irrespective of the mode of access, whether by laparotomy (6) or by laparoscopy (21), because it results in an anterior suspension of the uterus which increases the patient's subsequent risk of developing a rectocele and/or enterocele (19). This was observed with the original "vaginal-isthmic-colpopexy" (6). But, this is certainly not the case with the technique we employ, which is a lateral and not an anterior suspension. It is also completely different from the classical round ligament anterior fixation. Furthermore, our technique includes treatment of the posterior compartment by the reattachment of the uterosacral ligaments with occlusion of the pouch of Douglas and the additional laparoscopic posterior colporrhaphy. Finally, when necessary, to improve the support of the inferior part of the posterior vaginal wall and reduce the vulvo-vaginal enlargement, we associate a perineorrhaphy to the procedure which is carried out by the vaginal route.

Although laparoscopic lateral utero-vaginal suspension permits the association of a hysterectomy (total or subtotal), the procedure is particularly indicated for women presenting predominantly with a uterine prolapse and cystocele and and who wish to have a conservative surgical treatment. In regard to laparoscopic sacrocolpopexy, the contraindications are severe pelvic and abdominal adhesions, usually secondary to iterative laparotomies for bowel surgery and pelvic peritonitis. Other absolute and/or relative contraindications include obesity, cardiac disease, and respiratory insufficiency. In such cases procedures that use vaginal access, and when necessary loco-regional anesthesia would be preferable. An obvious contraindication is limited experience on the part of the surgeon.

The authors look forward to the corroboration of our encouraging results by others, preferably through more extensive studies with respect to both numbers of patients and the duration of follow-up.

REFERENCES

1. Vancaillie TG, Schuessler W. Laparoscopic bladder neck suspension. J Laparoendosc Surg 1991; 1:169–75.
2. Nezhat CH, Nezhat F, Nezhat C. Laparoscopic sacral colpopexy for vaginal vault prolapse. Obstet Gynecol 1994; 84:885–8.
3. Dorsey JH, Cundiff G. Laparoscopic procedures for incontinence and prolapse. Curr. Opinion Obstet Gynecol 1994; 6:223–30.
4. Mahendran D, Prashar S, Smith ARB, Murphy D. Laparoscopic sacrocolpopexy in the management of vaginal vault prolapse. Gynaecol Endosc 1996; 5: 217–22.
5. Dubuisson JB, Chapron C. Laparoscopic iliac colpo-uterine suspension for treatment of genital prolapse using two meshes. A new operative technique. J Gynecol Surg 1998; 14:153–9.
6. Kapandji M. Cure des prolapsus uro-génitaux par colpo-isthmo-cystopexie par bandelettes transversales et la douglassoraphie ligamento-péritonéale étagée et croisée. Ann Chir 1967; 21:321–8.
7. Chapron C, Dubuisson JB, Aubert V, et al. Total laparoscopic hysterectomy preliminary results. Hum Reprod 1994; 9:2084–9.
8. Bump RC, Mattiasson A, Brubaker LP, et al. The standardization of terminology of female pelvic organ prolapse and pelvic floor dysfonction. Am J Obstet Gynecol 1996; 175:10–17.
9. Dubuisson JB, Chapron C, Fauconnier A, Babaki-Fard K, Dendrinos S. Laparoscopic management of genital prolapse: lateral suspension with two meshes. Gynaecol Endosc 2000; 9:363–8.
10. Walsh DJ, Liu CY. Laparoscopic vaginal vault suspension (high McCall procedure): a review of 55 cases. Gynaecol Endosc 1997; 6:35.
11. Lam A, Rosen D. A new laparoscopic approach for enterocele repair. Gynaecol Endosc 1997; 6:211–17.
12. Vancaillie TG. Laparoscopic colposuspension and pelvic floor repair. Curr Opin Obstet Gynecol 1997; 9:244–6.
13. Wattiez A, Canis M, Alexandre F, et al. Laparoscopic approach to total pelvic prolapse. J Am Ass Gynecol Laparosc 1995; 2:59–63.
14. De Lancey JO. Anatomic aspects of vaginal eversion after hysterectomy. Am J Obstet Gynecol 1992; 166:1717–24.
15. Hardiman PJ, Drutz HP. Sacrospinous vault suspension and abdominal colpo sacropexy: success rates and complications. Am J Obstet Gynecol 1996; 175: 612–16.

16. Sutton GP, Addison WA, Livengood CH, Hammond CB. Life threatening hemorrage complicating sacral colpopexy. Am J Obstet Gynecol 1981; 140: 836–7.
17. Valaitis SR, Stanton SL. Sacrocolpopexy: a retrospective study of a clinician's experience. Br J Obstet Gynaecol 1994; 101:518–22.
18. Lefranc JP, Blondon J, Robert AHG. Chirurgie des prolapsus génitaux par voie abdominale. Expérience de la clinique chirurgicale et gynécologique de la Salpêtrière. J Chir (Paris); 1983; 120:401–6.
19. Hoff J, Manelfe A, Portet A, Giraud C. Promontofixation ou suspension par bandelette transversale? Etude comparée de ces deux techniques dans le traitement des prolapsus génitaux. Ann Chir 1984; 38:363–7.
20. Rimailho J, Talbot C, Bernard JD, Hoff J, Becue J. L'hystéropexie antéro-latérale par voie abdominale. Résultats et indications. A propos d'une série de quatre-vingt- douze patients. Ann Chir 1993; 47:244–9.
21. Cornier E, Madelenat P, Hysteropexie selon M. Kapandji. Technique per-coelioscopique et résultats préliminaires. J Gynecol Obstet Biol Reprod 1994; 23:378–85.

14

Lateral Sidewall Defects: Diagnosis and Treatment

Thomas Lyons

*Department of Obstetrics and Gynecology, Emory University,
Atlanta, Georgia, U.S.A.*

Defects of the anterior wall appear to be the best understood of the pelvic floor support defects. Despite this fact there are still over 300 methods described for treatment of these defects making our understanding of the pathophysiology of this area somewhat suspect. Still, at this point in surgical history it is reasonable to say that there are "gold standards" in the treatment of urinary stress incontinence (USI).

Most uro-gynecologists would agree that with anterior wall mobility a Burch retro-pubic culpo-suspension or a sub-urethral sling procedure would be the procedure of choice for USI in this group of patients. The type of sub-urethral sling [tension-free vaginal tape (TVT) versus transobturator tape (TOT)] certainly might be debated but this is more of a matter of surgeon preference than an actual difference in anatomic effect.

At the same time, if the patient has significant other defects, i.e., cystocele, enterocele, or rectocele a differing approach may be necessary. The cystocele defect is most often caused by a separation of the vaginal endo-pelvic fascia from its natural insertion or attachment to the arcus tendinus fascia pelvis or White's line of the pelvis (Figs. 1 and 2). Rarely, there will be a midline defect in this fascial unit resulting in a midline cystocele or even at times an anterior enterocele defect causing a cystocele. More often, a lateral separation occurs resulting in unilateral or bilateral para-vaginal defects. These para-vaginal defects are best addressed using a site-specific repair with restoration of the fascial attachments. Complete repair of all defects will always give the patient the best chance of long-term success of the repair and positive clinical results.

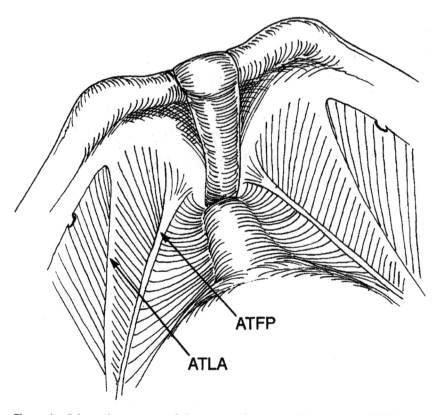

Figure 1 Schematic anatomy of the retropubic space. *Abbreviations*: ATFP, arcus tendineus fascia pelvis; ATLA, arcus tendineus levator ani.

There is some suggestion that a similar lateral wall attachment exists for the posterior floor, and standing magnetic resonance imaging studies on nulliparous patients have provided evidence that this is the case. However, this line of attachment has not been visualized in vivo and we must not assume that this is in fact an anatomic entity until more evidence is presented.

HISTORY

The history of surgical repair in this area dates to 1951 with the retropubic urethra-pexy, or Marshall-Marchetti-Krantz procedure. Although the procedure did not directly address lateral attachment defects, there were minor variations of this procedure that supposedly addressed the cystocele defect. In 1959 and later in 1961, Burch described his retropubic colposuspension, which began as a lateral attachment and then was changed into using the arcuate or Cooper's ligament structures as the site of reattachment.

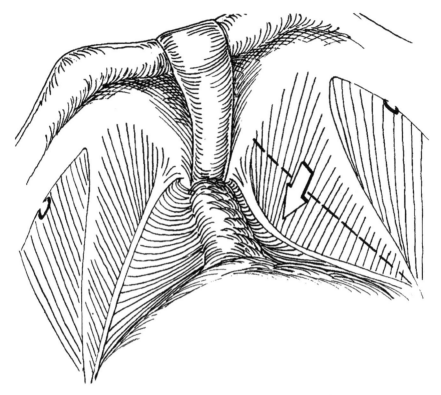

Figure 2 Schematic anatomy of paravaginal defect (*see arrow*).

Tanangho further modified the procedure to the accepted method used today. This procedure, in the current author's opinion acts predominately as a layering of the para-vaginal repair and thus constitutes a type of lateral wall defect repair.

Richardson et al. finally described the true para-vaginal repair with appropriate anatomic correlations in his milestone work in 1976. Richardson proposed either a vaginal or retro-pubic approach to these defects using the established arcus tendineus fascia pelvis and the arcus levator ani as attachment points for correction of the lateral wall defects. He further noted that the right para-vaginal defects were more common because more deliveries occur with the left occiput anterior presentation thus creating more stress to this right side of the pelvic wall.

Subsequently, Shull has described the para-vaginal plus procedure (para-vaginal repair plus Burch procedure) in the late 1980's and John Delancey has provided further anatomic foundation of these descriptions while coining the term "site specific" repair.

The latest chapters in this continually evolving story are in the area of application of minimally invasive techniques to the anatomic fundamentals espoused by Richardson, Delancey, and Shull. Early developers in this area have been Liu, Lyons, Wattiez, Miklos and others. It is of importance to note that the ability to access and visualize the anterior compartment in vivo, using laparoscopic techniques with their enlargement has provided surgeons with significant information regarding the anatomic and physiologic aspects of this area which was not available to the pioneers. Cadaver dissection although important was not as helpful as this in vivo view to the functional activities of the structures involved. It is also appropriate to include in this area the developers of the TVT and TOT procedures as, although these are predominately USI procedures, they still have an effect on the antero-lateral wall.

ANATOMY

Delancey has described the anterior compartment elegantly and classified the defects according to position and function. Figures 1 and 2 provide the reader with a perspective of this area anatomically with the defects that require treatment. Figures 3 and 4 provide a laparoscopic view in vivo of the retro-pubic space and the defects to be repaired.

TECHNIQUE

The description provided here will be that of the laparoscopic approach to lateral wall defects. The repair accomplished via laparotomy is identical but performed via a low transverse (Pfannenstiel) incision with entry into the space of Retsius using a pre-peritoneal approach. With the open

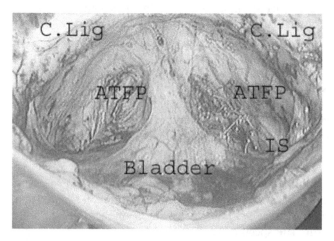

Figure 3 Laparoscopic anatomy of the retropubic space. *Abbreviation*: IS, ischial spine.

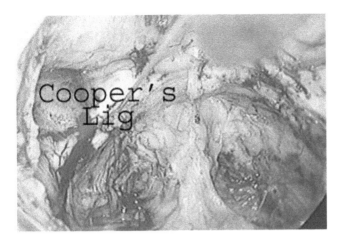

Figure 4   Laparoscopic view of retropubic space and paravaginal defects.

laparotomy, visualization of anatomic landmarks can be more difficult and accurate placement of sutures may be compromised.

Laparoscopically, the space of Retzius may be entered using a pre-peritoneal approach or a trans-peritoneal approach. In the pre-peritoneal approach, an open laparoscopy technique is recommended with entry down to the posterior sheath of the rectus fascia. The trocar is then anchored after gentle blunt dissection of this space and the pneumoperitoneum is allowed to complete the dissection into the space. The laparoscope itself is used as a blunt dissector, or at times a balloon cannula or an optically guided trocar can be used to facilitate this dissection. Secondary trocars are placed then under direct visualization to prepare for the repair. This technique is fast but often does not provide as good a look at the lateral wall area near the ischial spines and therefore is not used in our clinic. Furthermore, most patients with paravaginal defects will have posterior wall defects that will need to be repaired; these repairs should be done first, making the pre-peritoneal approach impossible laproscopically.

The standard trocar placement for this repair is shown in Figure 5. Posterior repairs and other ancillary procedures (hysterectomy, etc.) are completed prior to approaching the anterior compartment. An incision is made one inch above the symphysis pubis (identified by palpation) or the bladder can be filled with saline temporarily until the space can be identified. The incision is extended laterally to the obliterated umbilical ligaments and slightly caudad toward the symphysis. Blunt dissection carries the operator into the space. Anatomic landmarks are visualized (symphysis, Cooper's ligaments, obturator, neurovascular canal and the neurovascular bundle, ischial spines, arcus tendineus fascia pelvis, vaginal endopelvic fascia,

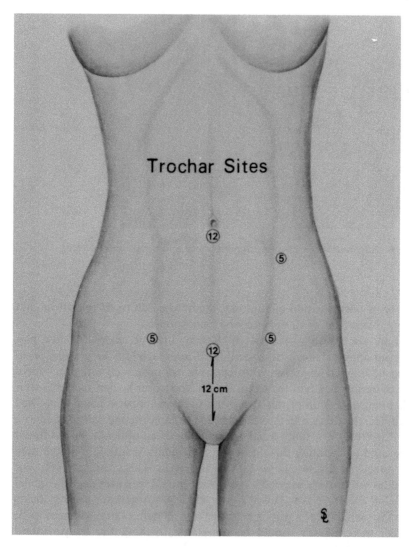

Figure 5 Trochar sites.

bladder, urethra) At this point after cleaning the structure of fat or areolar tissue the paravaginal defect should be visualized (Figs. 6 and 7). This defect is then closed using nonabsorbable sutures. This can be done using interrupted sutures or a variation of a running stitch. The initial suture should be placed close to the ischial spine on the lateral wall as this is the deepest point in the pelvis and will be the first obscured if any bleeding occurs during the suturing process (Fig. 8). The vaginal endo-pelvic fascia is reattached to the arcus with a suture until the defect is closed. After bilateral repair of the para-vaginal defect

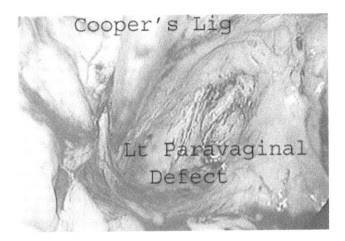

Figure 6 Laparoscopic view of left paravaginal defect.

(if necessary), the Burch procedure is then performed placing ten non-absorbable sutures on each side 1 to 2 cm lateral to the urethra into the endo-pelvic fascia using a figure-of-eight pass and then through Cooper's ligament, further stabilizing the anterior wall and correcting the antero-lateral wall defects. These sutures are placed first at the mid-urethral site and then at the urethra-vesical (UV) junction. Burch sutures should not be placed above this UV junction lest a funneling effect be caused, creating greater tendency for USI (Figs. 9 and 10).

After completion of the "paravaginal plus" procedure in the laparoscopic approach, the operator can easily inspect the vaginal vault, and,

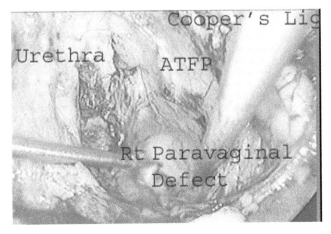

Figure 7 Laparoscopic view of right paravaginal defect.

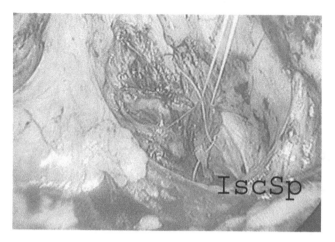

Figure 8   Suture placed to repair right paravaginal defect.

because there is increased intra-abdominal pressure due to the pneumo-peritoneum, the surgeon can evaluate the success of the repair. If the defects seem corrected, cystoscopy is performed to document ureteral patency as well as the absence of suture material in the bladder. If this inspection is negative then the anterior wall peritoneum is closed with a 2-0 polyglycolic acid suture placed in a purse-string fashion. If the procedure is performed using a laparotomy or in any pre-peritoneal approach of course there is no peritoneal defect to repair. Of course, it is critical to assure that haemostasis is achieved prior to closure and most operators, who perform the procedure

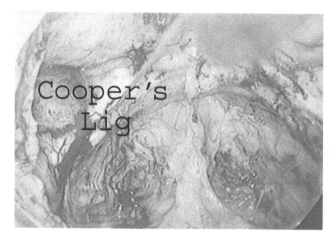

Figure 9   Right paravaginal defect repaired.

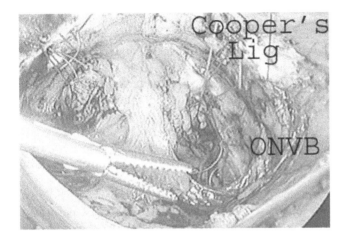

Figure 10 Burch sutures placed. *Abbreviation*: ONVB, obturator neurovascular bundle.

via laparotomy, will leave a drain in the space of Retsius for 72 hours post-operatively.

The choice of bladder drainage post-operatively is quite variable. Some surgeons chose a supra-pubic catheter versus a Foley. In our laparoscopic procedures, we use a Foley catheter that is removed in the recovery room. The patient is allowed to attempt to void for 5 hours after removal of the catheter and if unsuccessful the catheter is replaced overnight. In all patients the catheter is removed in the subsequent morning and if necessary the patient is taught intermittent self catheterization. Well over 90% of the patients are voiding spontaneously on the day of surgery and significantly less than one percent of patients require self catheter training. This reflects the fact that the procedure is performed in a less obstructive fashion with no intention to create an overly acute urethro-vesical angle with the Burch sutures.

It should also be noted that the para-vaginal repair can be performed without the Burch procedure and a sub-urethral sling (TVT or TOT) substituted if this is the operators standard. Both the TVT and the TOT are complimentary and seem to be equally effective in current data on USI.

Patients are required to observe pelvic rest for 6 to 8 weeks post-operatively. Repetitive straining or heavy lifting must be avoided for this same period. The patient can return to all other normal activities limited only by post-operative pain and other routine limitations.

DISCUSSION

Pelvic floor reconstruction is definitely a work in progress. With that being said it is this current author's opinion that we are closer to the finished product in the area of the anterior wall than in most of the other areas of the pelvis. The anatomy and physiology of this area appear to be a known although there is still some speculation of the exact continence mechanism. Lateral wall attachments are defined and have been since Richardson described them in 1976. Fascial support here appears to be well understood. In that regard the para-vaginal repair remains the gold standard for the repair of these defects. Most cystoceles are the result of lateral wall fascial separation at the level of the arcus tendineus fascia pelvis. Much less common are midline fascial breaks or the "anterior enterocele" defect allowing the bladder to herniate around the vault apex. Site specific correction of these defects seems to be the appropriate solution.

The only question therefore is not whether to repair but how to repair. Certainly these repairs can be made using traditional laparotomy techniques but today the ability to make the repairs effectively using lower morbidity laparoscopically guided procedures can be a great service to the patients.

It is imperative that these patients be encouraged to limit repetitive stress activities as frequently the post-operative recovery is very rapid and patients will have a tendency to do "too much". Also, the development and use of new graft and suture materials may be appropriate in some cases so the evolution of repairs in this area is continuing. Unfortunately, at times it takes several years to assess the real validity and morbidity of any new technique or device so knowing what is best in any given situation can be difficult. Suffice to say that any surgeon who works in the area of pelvic floor reconstruction must be knowledgeable, versatile, resourceful, and resilient if he or she is to be successful at treating these pervasive problems.

BIBLIOGRAPHY

Bergman A, Ballard CA, Konings PP. Comparison of three different surgical procedures for genuine stress incontinence: prospective randomized study. Am J Obstet Gynecol 1989; 160:1102—7.

Burch JC. Cooper's ligament urethro-vesical suspension for urinary stress incontinence. Am J Obstet Gynecol 1968; 100:764–71.

Burch JC. Urethro-vaginal fixation to Cooper's ligament for correction of stress incontinence, cystocele, and prolapse. Am J Obstet Gynecol 1961; 81:281–6.

Burton GA. A randomized comparison of laparoscopic and open colpo-suspension. Neurol Urodyn 1994; 13:487–98.

Burton GA. A three-year randomized urodynamic study comparing open and laparoscopic colposuspension. Neurol Urodynam 1997; 16:353–4.

Cooper MJW, Cario G, Lam A, Carlton M. A review of results in a series of 113 laparoscopic colpo-suspensions. Aust NZ J Obst Gynec 1996; 36:44–8.

Das S. Comparative outcome analysis of laparoscopic colposuspension, abdominal colposuspension and vaginal needle suspension for female urinary incontinence. J Urol 1998; 160:368–71.

Demco L. Hysterectomy panel discussion. J Am Assoc Gynecol Laparosc 1994; 13: 287–95.

Fatthy H, El Hao M, Samaha I, Abdallah K. Modified Burch colposuspension: laparoscopy versus laparotomy. J Am Assoc Gynecol Laparosc 2001; 8:99–106.

Gittes RF. No incision pubo-vaginal suspension for stress incontinence. J Urol 1987; 138:568–74.

Gunn GC, Cooper RP, Gordon NS, Gagnon L. Use of a new device for endoscopic suturing in the laparoscopic Burch procedure. J Am Assoc Gynecol Laparosc 1994; 2:65–70.

Kelly HA. Incontinence of urine in women. Uro Certan Rev 1913; 17:291–9.

Kreder KJ, Winfield HN. Laparoscopic urethral sling for treatment of intrinsic sphincter deficiency. J Endourol 1996; 10:255–7.

Kung RC, Lie K, Lee P, Drutz HP. The cost effectiveness of laparoscopic versus abdominal Burch in women with urinary stress incontinence. J Am Assoc Gynecol Laparosc 1996; 3:537–44.

Lam AM, Jenkins GJ, Hyslop RS. Laparoscopic Burch colpo-suspension for stress incontinence: preliminary results. Med J Aust 1995; 162:18–21.

Langebrekke A, Dahlstrom B, Eraker R, Urnes A. The laparoscopic Burch procedure. A preliminary report. Acta Obstet Gynecol Scand 1995; 74:153–5.

Lee CL, Yen CF, Wang CJ, Huang KG, Soong YK. Extraperitoneal colposuspension using CO2 distension method. Int Surg 1998; 83:262–4.

Lee CL, Yen CF, Wang CJ, Jain S, Soong YK. Extraperitoneal approach to laparoscopic Burch colposuspension. J Am Assoc Gynecol Laparosc 2001; 8: 374–7.

Leissner J, Allhoff EF, Naumann G, et al. Inguinovaginal sling procedure for female stress incontinence: introduction of a minimally invasive technique. Tech Urol 2001; 7:105–9.

Levy BS, Hulka JS, Peterson HB, et al. Operative Laparoscopy: AAGL membership survey. J Am Assoc Gynecol Laparosc 1994; 14:301–14.

Liu CY. Laparoscopic retro-pubic colpo-suspension (Burch procedure). A review of 58 cases. J Reprod Med 1993; 38:526–30.

Liu CY. Laparoscopic treatment of genuine urinary stress incontinence. Baillieres Clin Obstet Gynaecol 1994; 8:789–98.

Liu CY, Paek W. Laparoscopic retro-pubic colpo-suspension (Burch procedure). J Am Assoc Gynecol Laparosc 1993; 1:31–5.

Lobel RW, Davis GD. Long-term results of laparoscopic Burch urethro-pexy. J Am Assoc Gynecol Laparosc 1997; 4:341–5.

Lyons TL. Minimally invasive retro-pubic colpo-suspension. Gynaecol Endosc 1995; 4:189–94.

Lyons TL. Minimally invasive treatment of urinary stress incontinence and laparoscopically directed repair of pelvic floor defects. Clin Obstet Gynecol 1995; 38:380–91.

Lyons TL, Winer WK. Clinical outcomes with laparoscopic approaches and open Burch procedures for urinary stress incontinence. J Am Assoc Gynecol Laparosc 1995; 2:193–8.

Margossian H, Walters MD, Falcone T. Laparoscopic management of pelvic organ prolapse. Eur J Obstet Gynecol Reprod Biol 1999; 85:57–62.

Marshall VF, Marchetti AA, Krantz KE. The correction of stress incontinence by simple vesicourethral suspension. Surg Gynecol Obstet 1949; 88:590.

Miannay E, Cosson M, Lanvin D, Querleu D, Crepin G. Comparison of open retropubic and laparoscopic colposuspension for treatment of urinary stress incontinence. Eur J Obstet Gynecol Reprod Biol 1998; 79:159–66.

Miklos JR, Kohli N. Laparoscopic para-vaginal repair plus Burch urethro-pexy: review and descriptive technique. Urol 2000; 56:64–9.

Narepalem N, Kreder KJ, Winfield HN. Laparoscopic urethral sling for the treatment of intrinsic urethral weakness (type III urinary stress incontinence). Tech Urol Vol 1995; 1:102–5.

Nezhat CH, Nezhat F, Nezhat CR, Rottenberg H. Laparoscopic retro-pubic cysto-urethropexy. J Am Assoc Gynecol Laparosc 1994; 1:339–49.

Nichols DH, Ponchak SF. Treating incontinence transvaginally. Cont Obstet Gynecol (Supplement) 1986; 109–21.

Nieves A. Long-term results of laparoscopic Burch. J Am Assoc Gynecol Laparosc 1996; 3:S35.

Papasakelariou C, Papasakelariou B. Laparoscopic bladder neck suspension. J Am Assoc Gynecol Laparosc 1997; 4:185–9.

Pereyra AS. A simplified procedure for correction of stress incontinence. J Surg Gynecol Obstet 1959; 67:223–6.

Polascik TJ, Moore RG, Rosenberg MT, Kavoussi LR. Comparison of laparoscopic and open retro-pubic urethro-pexy for treatment of urinary stress incontinence. Urology 1995; 45:647–52.

Radomski SB, Herschorn S. Laparoscopic Burch bladder neck suspension: early results. J Urol 1996; 155:515–18.

Raz S, Sussman FM, Erickson DB, Bugg KS, Nitti VW. The Raz bladder neck suspension results in 206 patients. J Urol 1992; 148:845–50.

Richardson AC, Edmonds PB, Williams N. Treatment of urinary stress incontinence due to para-vaginal fascial defect. Obstet Gynecol 1982; 57:357–60.

Ridley JH. Appraisal of the Goebell-Frangenheim-Stoeckel sling procedure. Am J Obstet Gynecol 1966; 95:714–21.

Ross J. Two techniques of laparoscopic Burch repair for stress incontinence: a prospective, randomized study. J Am Assoc Gynecol Laparosc 1996; 3:351–7.

Ross JW. Multichannel urodynamic evaluation of laparoscopic Burch colposuspension for genuine stress incontinence. Obstet Gynecol 1998; 91:55–9.

Saidi MH, Sadler RK, Saidi JA. Extraperitoneal laparoscopic colposuspension for genuine urinary stress incontinence. J Am Assoc Gynecol Laparosc 1998; 5: 247–52.

Shull BL. Anterior paravaginal defects. In TeLinde's Operative Gynecology, Philadelphia: Lippincott 1997:1006–30.

Shull BL. Anterior paravaginal defects. TeLinde's Operative Gynecology, Philadelphia: Lippincott. 1997:1006–30.

Shwayder JM. Laparoscopic Burch cysto-urethropexy compared with the transperitoneal and extraperitoneal approaches. J Am Assoc Gynecol Laparosc 1996; 3: S46–7.

Stamey TA. Endoscopic suspension of the vesicle neck for urinary incontinence in females: A report on 203 consecutive patients. Am Surg 1980; 192:465–71.

Su TH, Wang KG, Hsu CY, Wei HJ, Hong BK. Prospective comparison of laparoscopic and traditional colposuspensions in the treatment of genuine stress incontinence. Acta Obstet Gynecol Scand 1997; 76:576–82.

Vancaillie TG, Schuessler W. Laparoscopic bladder neck suspension. J Laparosc Endosc Surg 1991; 1:169–73.

von Theobald P, Guillaumin D, Levy G. Laparoscopic pre-peritoneal colpo-suspension for stress incontinence in women. Technique and results of 37 procedures. Surg Endosc 1995; 9:1189–92.

Wattiez A, Boughizane S, Alexandre F, Canis M, Mage G, Pouly JL, et al. Laparoscopic procedures for stress incontinence and prolapse. Curr Opin Obstet Gynecol 1995; 7:317–21.

Zacharin RF. The anatomic supports of the female urethra. Obstet Gynecol 1968; 32:754–9.

Zullo F, Palomba S, Piccione F, Morelli M, Arduino B, Mastrantonio P. Laparoscopic Burch colposuspension: a randomized controlled trial comparing two transperitoneal surgical techniques. Obstet Gynecol 2001; 98:783–8.

Part 4: The Posterior Segment

15

The Classical Techniques for Rectocele Repair: Complications and Outcome

P. Mendes da Costa

Department of Digestive and Endoscopic Surgery, CHU Brugmann, Université Libre de Bruxelles, Brussels, Belgium

Robrecht Van Hee

Academic Surgical Center Stuivenberg, ZNA Stuivenberg, University of Antwerp, Antwerp, Belgium

Christian Ngongang

Department of Digestive and Endoscopic Surgery, CHU Brugmann, Université Libre de Bruxelles, Brussels, Belgium

INTRODUCTION

Rectocele, a rectal hernia through the rectovaginal wall into the vagina, can be an important and disabling disease, often requiring surgical treatment. Rectoceles develop due to loosening of the normally strong interstitial connective tissue between vagina and rectum, mostly as the result of repeated and strong pressure exerted on the rectovaginal septum during labor, delivery, or forceful defecation.

Rectoceles are mostly asymptomatic but may induce a sensation of incomplete defecation due to filling of the herniated rectum with feces. Sometimes the hernial sac may descend outside the vagina and cause discomfort or even erosion of the prolapsing posterior vaginal wall.

Surgical treatment is indicated whenever symptoms of disabling defecation or vaginal discomfort occur. Many surgical treatments have been proposed since the earliest reports of posterior colporrhaphy. Different types of surgical approach may be used, either transvaginal, transanal, transperineal or transabdominal (1,2).

All these operation routes bear their own type and frequency of complications.

COMPLICATIONS

Transvaginal repair aims at restoration of the pelvic floor by suturing the levator ani muscles anteriorly to the rectum, combined with excision of redundant flaps of posterior vaginal wall (Figs. 1–4). One out of 10 vaginal interventions may be followed by hemorrhage, injury of the rectum or other adjacent organs, infection, or urinary retention. In the long term the vaginal approach may induce dyspareunia, rectovaginal fistula (5%), recurrent herniation or rectal sphincter dysfunction.

Transanal repair has been performed in several ways. At first inverting of redundant and prolapsing rectal tissue was realized by intraluminal reefing of the rectal wall.

This transanal procedure may bear different complications: hemorrhage has been recorded in 7%, endorectal suture dehiscence in 5%, distal stenosis in 2% and rectovaginal fistula in 1.5%. Anal dilatation, needed for the intervention, can induce sphincter injury, particularly when the perineum had previously been traumatised or partially denervated.

Recently a double stapling technique had been proposed (the STARR procedure) to achieve the rectal hernia closure: a double circumferential full

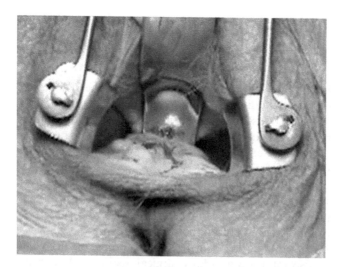

Figure 1 After exposure of the site a straight antero posterior incision is made with a no. 23 blade. The full thickness of the vaginal wall is transected to expose the underlying fascia.

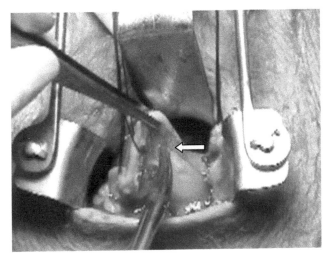

Figure 2   The full thickness vaginal wall is elevated and pulled to the sides to expose the enterocele. Further dissection is carried out as the forceps expose the tissues to the scissors. Note how closely the enterocele (*white arrow*) is located to the vaginal fascia.

thickness resection of the lower rectum is thereby realized, not only on the anterior prolapsing side, but also of the posterior rectal wall.

Also this type of transanal hernia correction may be followed by hemorrhage requiring readmission (4.4%), as well as by urinary retention

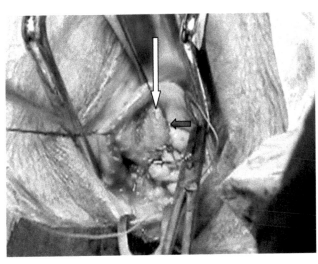

Figure 3   After approximation of the levator muscles (*white arrow*) the vaginal wall is secured first to the left with interrupted stitches Vicryl 0 (*small black arrow*).

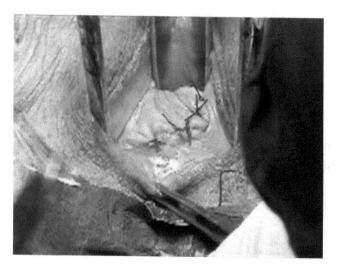

Figure 4   After securing both the vaginal wound edges, these are joined one to the other in the midline at the end of the intervention.

(5.6%). Mid-term complications include feeling of fecal urgency (17.8%), incontinence for flatus (8.9%), or late stenosis (3.3%).

Combined Vaginal and Transanal Approach

Some investigators have used a combined approach of both vaginal and transanal interventions. Van Dam et al. (3) analyzed the results of such approach in 89 patients. A successful outcome was obtained in 71% of patients. Previous hysterectomy did not seem to influence the results in this series.

Transperineal Route of Repair

D'Hoore (4) studied the long-term results in a series of 71 patients, who were operated upon with this kind of repair. They observed complete disappearance of dyschesia in 70% of their cases and an improvement of incomplete evacuation in 60% of the series. There was no dyspareunia in their series.

In a prospective study of Lechaux et al. (5), results of a series of transperineally operated patients were discussed. The success rate was 80%, while poor results were obtained in 9% of the patients. Clinical and manometric signs of anal hyperactivity proved to be correlated with poorer results.

Ayabaca et al. (6) published their results of a combined approach of transperineal and endorectal repair in a series of 60 patients with a median follow-up of 48 months; they noted good results in 73.5% of the cases and a recurrence rate of 10%.

Transabdominal Repair

This repair may either be performed by laparotomy or by laparoscopy. The operation generally consists of a polyglactin mesh fixation of the mobilized and raised rectum at the sacral promontory, and thereby parallels the surgical treatment of rectal prolapse (7). The transabdominal route has particularly been recommended when the rectocele is associated with an elytrocele (8).

Complications of such procedures have included prosthetic mesh infection, nerve injury, and mesh erosion into rectum or vagina. Most investigations now favor the laparoscopic approach (9). Some even have tried robotic assisted laparoscopy in high-grade vault prolapse (10). Complications of laparoscopic techniques equal those of open surgery, but avoid large incisions and accompanying drawbacks.

In a multicentric report from Italian colo-proctologists entitled "Which Surgical Approach for Rectocele," Boccasanta et al. (1) studied 2,212 patients. They observed 7.8% of hemorrhage, 5% of suture dehiscence, 2.1% of distal rectal stenosis, 1.4% of rectovaginal fistula, 16.4% of delayed healing of perineal wound, and 17% of dyspareunia.

Sullivan et al. (11) analyzed their 10-year experience in a series of 236 patients after total pelvic mesh repair. They observed an overall satisfaction rate of 74% after more than 6 years of follow-up. In a nonrandomized study, Grandjean et al. (8) compared the abdominal management of rectocele and elytrocele by laparotomy (37 patients) and by laparoscopic approach (35 patients); the results were an improvement in anal incontinence in 95% of all cases, an improvement of dyschesia in 80% of the cases and a recurrence rate of 3%. Laparoscopic approach seemed to be superior in terms of morbidity and functional results.

In conclusion, literature gives no clear response to the question of which surgical procedure to choose; the subject remains very controversial. There are too few comparative data in literature and failure and/or recurrence rates are highly variable. Moreover, there is no correlation between anatomic results and patient's complaints. Precise preoperative assessment is required and there is probably a place for dynamic MRI.

The complex anatomical and functional abnormalities should be taken into account, whether or not isolated or associated with other pelvic floor disorders. Surgeons should thereby be familiar with the various surgical procedures, in order to adapt their treatment according to the actual situation. Finally, a very long-term follow-up is necessary to evaluate the final results.

REFERENCES

1. Boccasanta P, Venturi M, Calabro G, et al. Which surgical approach for rectocele? A multicentric report from Italian coloproctologists. Tech Coloproctol 2001; 5:149–56.
2. Hager T. Chirurgische operationsverfahren zur therapie der rektozele. Visceral-chirurgie 2006; 41:196–201.
3. Van Dam JH, Hop WC, Schouten WR. Analysis of patients with poor outcome of rectocele repair. Dis Colon Rectum 2000; 43:1556–60.
4. D'Hoore A. Symptomatic outcome after transperineal rectocele repair: longterm results in 71 patients. Oral abstract, European Association of Coloproctology, Maastricht, 2001.
5. Lechaux JP, Lechaux D, Bataille P, Bars I. Transperineal repair of rectocele with prosthetic mesh. A prospective study. Ann Chir 2004; 129:211–17.
6. Ayabaca SM, Zbar AP, Pescatori M. Anal continence after rectocele repair. Dis Colon Rectum 2002; 45:63–9.
7. Ruppert M, Van Hee R, Hendrickx L, Creve U. Laparoscopic rectopexy for complete rectal prolapse. Min Invas Ther. Allied Technol 1996; 5:471–2.
8. Grandjean JP, Seket B, Galaup JP, et al. Abdominal management of rectocele and elytrocele: place of the laparoscopic approach. Ann Chir 2004; 129:87–93.
9. Lyons TL, Winer WK. Laparoscopic rectocele repair using polyglactin mesh. J Am Assoc Gynecol Laparosc 1997; 4:381–4.
10. Elliot D, Frank I, DiMarco D, Chow G. Gynecologic use of robotically assisted laparoscopy: Sacrocolpopexy for the treatment of high-grade vaginal vault prolapse. Am J Surg 2004; 188:52–6.
11. Sullivan ES, Longaker CJ, Lee P. Total pelvic mesh repair: a ten year experience. Dis. Colon Rectum 2001; 44:857–63.

16

Endoscopic Treatment of Elytrocele

Toon P. M. Sonneville

Endoscopic Gastrointestinal Surgery, Academic Surgical Center, Antwerp, Belgium

Descent of the posterior compartment induces a variety of pathologies: solitary rectal ulcer, recto-rectal intussusception, deep pouch of Douglas with elytrocele, rectal prolapse with or without incontinence, and in the female rectocele.

SURGICAL TECHNIQUE

The technique described herein is a rectopexy using an anterior mesh. It is our favorite technique because of the low incidence of postoperative-induced obstructive defecation and also because the procedure allows an easy treatment of the vaginal vault prolapse or uterine descent by colpopexy.

PRINCIPLES

There are different entities causing the pathology:

1. insufficient posterior fixation of rectum,
2. excessively deep pouch of Douglas,
3. weakening of the rectovaginal septum, and
4. diastases of the levator muscles.

Regarding the different theories concerning the pathogenesis of the condition, we cannot state the causes or the consequences in an absolute way.

HISTORICAL NOTE ON RECTOPEXY

1. *The posterior rectopexy without mesh*: Here the posterior aspect of the rectum is dissected, and the rectal wings are attached to the promontory, the technique can be associated with a sigmoidectomy (1).
2. *The posterior rectopexy with mesh (1,3–5)*: This technique causes a newly induced postoperative defecation problem in 50% of the patients. The etiology varies: kinking of the rectum, denervation, fibrosis and strangulation of the same.
3. *The anterior rectopexy with two individual prosthesis Orr-Loygue (6–8)*: This technique yields better results but because of the circular position of the prostheses some patients experience a degree of dyschezia. Therefore, Dulucq (9) proposed an early modification by positioning two prosthesis on each side of the rectum instead of around the organ.

MATERIALS NECESSARY FOR THE TECHNIQUE DESCRIBED

1. One optical trocar
2. One trocar highcap 12 mm reduction to 10 for the optical system in a left (5 cm) para-umbilical position
3. Hopkins rodlens scope of 10 mm (0 and 30 degrees have to be available)
4. Cold light fountain
5. Endoscopic camera
6. Two 5 mm trocars
    a. One suprapubic for an ancillary instrument
    b. One 2 cm above the left anterior superior spine
7. One trocar 10 to 12 mm umbilical for right hand instrument, the optical trocar can be used
8. Two atraumatic graspers
9. One pair of endoscopic scissors
10. One fixation device: stapler or "tacker"
11. One laparoscopic needle holder (the author prefers a 10 mm laparoscopic needle holder)
12. One vaginal probe; a sponge holder can be used instead
13. One rectal probe; Hegar or "drumstick" from the circular stapler
14. One CO_2 insufflator or abdominal wall lifting system
15. One polypropylene mesh

Positioning of the Patient

1. A classical colorectal preparation, common for all colorectal surgery, is used. One dose of prophylactic antibiotics is given during the induction

of the anesthesia. The patient is intubated and positioned in a dorsal decubitus with the legs in the gynecological position.

2. An indwelling bladder catheter is used.
3. The operation table is maneuvered in a 30° Trendelenburg position after the placement of the optical trocar.
4. The surgeon stands on the left of the patient.
5. The first assistant stands farther to the left of the surgeon.
6. The second assistant stands between the legs of the patient.
7. The video monitor is positioned at the right foot of the patient.

PNEUMOPERITONEUM AND POSITIONING OF THE TROCARS

1. A pneumoperitoneum of 16 mm Hg is created after accessing the peritoneal cavity with an optical trocar in the umbilicus. In the hands of the author this technique proves to be faster than the open Hasson access and safer than the Veress approach.
2. A second trocar (12 reduction to 10) is placed 5 cm para-umbilical to the left for the final position of the optic.
3. A 5 mm trocar at the inner side of the anterior superior iliac spine 2 cm higher
4. A 5 mm trocar suprapubic
5. If necessary a fourth trocar can be placed at the inner side of then right anterior superior iliac spine.

EXPOSITION OF RECTO SIGMOID

1. The patient is positioned in a 30 degree Trendelenburg.
2. The small bowel is retracted towards the cranial part of the abdominal cavity.
3. In the female patient if necessary a transparietal suture through the uterus brings the latter out of the operative field and can be used to give anterior traction during the suturing of the mesh on the rectum.
4. The pouch of Douglas is examined and the thickness of the para rectal peritoneum, caused by the descent, is evaluated.
5. The first incision is made at the right side on the peritoneum at the recto- sigmoidal junction.
6. The peritoneal incision is continued towards the deepest point and there extended from right to left.
7. In the female patient the application of a vaginal probe in the posterior fornix and one in the rectum facilitates the exposure of the rectovaginal septum (Fig. 1).

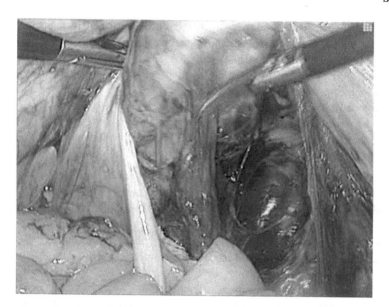

Figure 1 The forceps elevate the vagina, making the preparation of the rectum anterior wall easier. The probe in the rectum cannot be seen but helps to open the recto-vaginal septum.

THE RECTAL DISSECTION

In our technique only the anterior rectal wall is dissected free, from the vagina in the female and the Denonvilliers fascia in male, until the dissection reaches the level of the levator muscles.

In the female the anterior rectal wall is easier defined with help of a rectal probe and a vaginal probe in the posterior fornix moved in the antero-posterior axis of the pelvis in opposite directions.

Conserving all the latero-posterior rectal relations we believe to be able to avoid postoperative defecation disturbances, disturbances that occur in 50% of the posterior rectopexies.

The depth of dissection is checked under both visual (the probe in the rectum) and digital (the second assistants finger) control until 4 to 6 cm from the anal border.

DISSECTION OF THE PROMONTORY

After opening the peritoneum at the rectosigmoidal junction, further dissection is carried out posterior into the mesorectum above the promontory. An avascular area of $1\,cm^2$ is sufficient with respect to the middle sacral artery and the iliac vein and artery.

FIXATION OF THE PROSTHESIS

Rectal Fixation of the Prosthetic Tape

1. A mesh of 4 × 20 cm is introduced through the 12 mm trocar.
2. The mesh is sutured to the anterior rectal wall with zero-muscular stitches of 2/0 resorbable thread between four and six knots are used to fix the mesh to the anterior aspect of the rectum (Figs. 2–5).

Positioning of the Tape

The tape is positioned at the right side of the rectum. Because by using this technique there is no encircling of the rectum no possibility is created to cause strangulation.

Anchoring the Mesh to the Promontory

1. The lumbosacral disc is freed over a small area, taking care of the right ureter and both the sacral and the iliac vessels, the spot on which we tacker or staple the mesh, without any kind of traction, the tape simply holds the rectum in place (Fig. 6).
2. Redundant prosthetic material is resected.

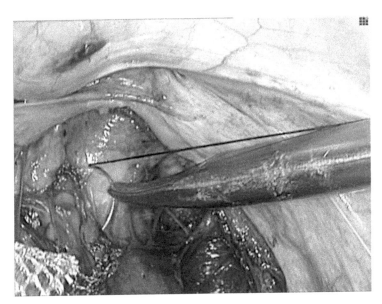

Figure 2 The prosthesis is introduced. The first stitch, which is placed in the middle some 1.5 cm from the levator ani as a serosa muscularis stitch.

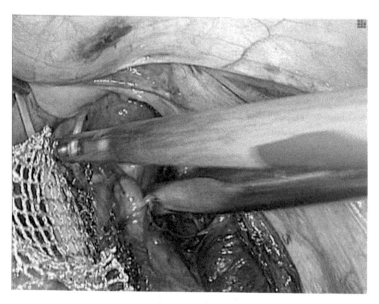

Figure 3 The second and third stitches are placed on the lateral anterior margin of the rectum.

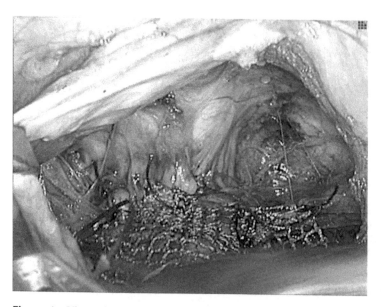

Figure 4 View of the distal part of the prosthesis. Note that the prosthesis is flattened out over the anterior aspect of the rectum.

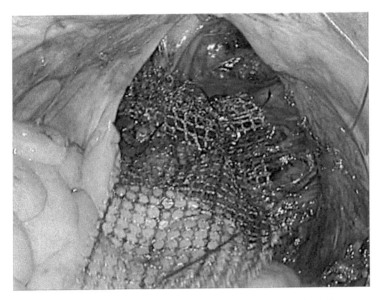

Figure 5 The final image after the securing of the prosthesis by two other lateral stitches.

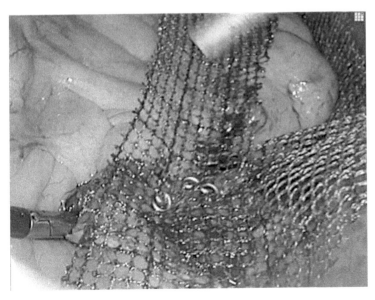

Figure 6 The proximal end of the prosthesis is now anchored in the free space, which has been dissected earlier on the anterior aspect of the last lumbar vertebra of the sacrum.

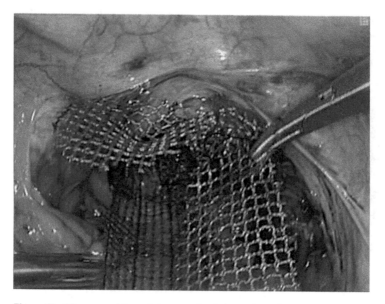

Figure 7 The second leg of the prosthesis is anchored onto the vagina elevated by a forceps to be in the operating field.

PERITONEALIZATION AND DOUGLASECTOMY

The reperitonealization is executed with a 2/0 resorbable thread. Excess peritoneal tissue in pouch of Douglas is resected or placated.

Associated Pathology

Genital Prolapse

A second tape can be sutured to the uterine isthmus and fixed to the promontory or less cumbersome, the isthmus can be sutured to the first tape. Here the author uses a Y shaped mesh fashioned during the operation to the needs of the pelvic area at hand (Fig. 7).

Then the reperitonealization and douglasectomy is carried out as described previously.

CONCLUSION

By using this technique the major causes for postoperative "de novo" defecation problems are avoided (10). The fact that the innervation of the rectum is spared during the dissection could well be the reason for the fact that no defecation problems were seen in the small sample of patients ($n = 11$) during a follow-up of 2 to 12 months. Further investigations are necessary to draw conclusions. The laparoscopic approach to treat the three compartments during one surgery is well tolerated by the patients (median age of 64 years). All but one patient left the hospital on day two postoperatively although the median duration of the intervention was of 4.30 hours (laparoscopic Burch colpopexy and subtotal hysterectomy included). No complications due to the prosthetic material or the laparoscopic technique have been recorded in the patients who underwent the technique.

ACKNOWLEDGMENTS

This technique was developed during the care of patients seen by the Pelvic Floor Task Force of ZNA STER Site Stuivenberg consisting of surgeons, urologists, gynecologists, radiologists, revalidations doctors, and gastro-enterologists. The operations were carried out with collaboration between surgeons and gynecologists.

REFERENCES

1. Frykman HM, Goldberg SM. The surgical treatment of rectal procidentia. Surg Gynecol Obstet 1969; 129(6):1225–30.
2. Ripstein CB. Procidentia: definitive corrective surgery. Dis Colon Rectum 1972; 15(5):334–6.
3. Wells C. New operation for rectal prolapse. Proc R Soc Med 1959; 52:602–3.
4. Himpens J, Cadiere BG, Bruybs J, Vertruyen M. Laparoscopic rectopexy according to Wells. Surg Endosc 1999; 13(2):139–41.
5. Morgan CN, Porter NH, Klugman DJ. Ivalon (polyvinyl alcohol) sponge in the repair of complete rectal prolapse. Br J Surg 1972; 59(II):841–6.
6. Portier G, Iovino F, Lazorthes F. Surgery for rectal prolapse: Orr-Logue ventral rectopexy with limited dissection prevents postoperative-induced constipation without increasing recurrence. Dis Colon Rectum 2006; 49(8): 1136–40.
7. Marchal F, Bresler L, Ayav A, et al. Long-term results of Delorme's procedure and Orr-Loygue rectopexy to treat rectal prolapse. Dis Colon Rectum 2005; 48 (9):1785–90.
8. Loygue J, Nordlinger B, Cunci O, Malafosse M, Huguet C, Parc R. Rectopexy to the promontory for the treatment of rectal prolapse. Report of 257 cases. Dis Colon Rectum 1984; 27(6):356–9.
9. Dulucq JL. Traîtement des prolapsus du rectum par laparoscopie. Encycl Méd Chir (Elsevier Paris) Techniques Chirurgicales—Appareil Digestif. 1998; 40: 711–17.
10. D'Hoore A, Cadoni R, Penninckx F. Long-term outcome of laparoscopic ventral rectopexy for total rectal prolapse. Br J Surg 2004; 91(11):1389.

Index